DRUGS AND THE LIVER:
HIGH RISK PATIENTS AND TRANSPLANTATION

Medical Science Symposia Series

Volume 4

The titles published in this series are listed at the end of this volume.

Drugs and the Liver: High Risk Patients and Transplantation

Edited by

D. Galmarini

Institute of Surgical Researches and Transplantation,
Ospedale Maggiore Policlinico di Milano,
University of Milan, Milan, Italy

L.R. Fassati

Institute of Surgical Researches and Transplantation,
Ospedale Maggiore Policlinico di Milano,
University of Milan, Milan, Italy

R. Paoletti

Institute of Pharmacological Sciences,
University of Milan, Milan, Italy

and

S. Sherlock

Royal Free Hospital School of Medicine,
University of London, London, U.K.

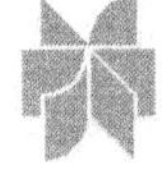

SPRINGER SCIENCE+BUSINESS MEDIA, B.V.

Library of Congress Cataloging-in-Publication Data

Drugs and the liver : high risk patients and transplantation / edited by D. Galmarini ... [et al.].
p. cm. -- (Medical science symposiaseries ; v.4)
Includes index.
ISBN 978-0-7923-2307-5 ISBN 978-94-011-1994-8 (eBook)
DOI 10.1007/978-94-011-1994-8
1. Liver--Transplantation--Complications--Congresses. 2. Liver--Effect of drugs on--Congresses. 3. Liver--Surgery--Risk factors--Congresses. 4. Cyclosporine--Physiological effect--Congresses. I. Galmarini, D. II. Series.
[DNLM: 1. Liver Transplantation--immunology--congresses. 2. Liver Diseases--drug therapy--congresses. 3. Immunosuppressive Agents--therapeutic use--congresses. 4. Graft Rejection--drug therapy--congresses. WI 770 D794 1993]
RD546.D78 1993
617.5'56--dc20
DNLM/DLC
for Library of Congress 93-1383

ISBN 978-0-7923-2307-5

Printed on acid-free paper

Contents

Preface

The **International Symposium on DRUGS AND THE LIVER: High Risk Patients and Transplantation** provided an international forum for the discussion of the different pharmacological and biochemical aspects of the clinical transplantation of the liver. The objective of the meeting was to focus discussion on the effects of the damage to the liver, the quality of the harvested organ, the antiblastic and immunosuppressive drugs used, and the results after hepatic transplantation in high-risk patients.

The goal of this volume is to present the findings on the current state of clinical and experimental research on hepatic pathology and the pathology of the liver. It is apparent from this body of knowledge that a need exists for the formulation of an interdisciplinary focus for all scientists involved in the problems of liver transplantation. The chapters here included are presented following the order of the scientific program of the symposium.

The organizers wish to thank each participant in this Symposium for the generous scientific input provided. We also gratefully acknowledge the device and aid provided by the staff of the Fondazione Giovanni Lorenzini, which ensured the smooth functioning of the meeting. We also appreciate the financial support by the sponsors that made this symposium and this publication possible and in particular our thanks go to A.I.R.C (Italian Association for Cancer Research), Sandoz Prodotti Farmaceutici S.p.A. and Cilag S.p.A..

The Editors

List of Contributors

M. Alessiani
Department of Surgery
University of Pittsburgh
School of Medicine
3601 Fifth Avenue
5C Falk Clinic
Pittsburgh, PA 15213
USA

G. Annoni
Istituto di Medicina Interna
Università degli Studi di Milano
Via Pace 9
20122 Milan
Italy

G. Antonelli
Institute of Virology
Viale di Porta Tiburtina 28
00185 Rome
Italy

B. Arosio
Istituto di Medicina Interna
Università degli Studi di Milano
Via Pace 9
20122 Milan
Italy

D. Azoulay
Service de Chirurgie Hépatobiliaire
Paul Brousse
94800 Villejuif
France

E. Beck
Istituto di Anestesia e Rianimazione dell'Università degli Studi
Ospedale Maggiore IRCCS Milano
Via F. Sforza 35
20122 Milan
Italy

T. Bienvenu
Laboratoire de Pharmacologie Périnatale et Pédiatrique
St Vincent de Paul
75014 Paris
France

H. Bismuth
Service de Chirurgie Hépatobiliaire
Paul Brousse
94800 Villejuif
France

J. Bleck
Abteilung Gastroenterologie und Hepatologie
Medizinische Hochschule Hannover
DW-3000 Hannover
Germany

L.P. Bonara
Centro Trapianto Fegato
Ospedale Maggiore IRCCS Milano
Istituto di Chirurgia Sperimentale e dei Trapianti
Università degli Studi
Via F. Sforza 35
20122 Milan
Italy

C.A. Brass
Gastrointestinal Section
University of Pennsylvania
School of Medicine
Philadelphia, PA 19104
USA

M. Burdelski
Kinderklinik
Medizinische Hochschule Hannover
DW-3000 Hannover 61
Germany

H. Burgmann
Institut für Medizinische Physiologie
University of Vienna
A-1090 Vienna
Austria

L. Caccamo
Centro Trapianto Fegato
Ospedale Maggiore IRCCS Milano
Istituto di Chirurgia Sperimentale
e dei Trapianti
Università degli Studi
Via F. Sforza 35
20122 Milan
Italy

P. Canioni
Laboratoire de RMN de l'IBCN-CNRS
Université de Bordeaux II
1, rue Camille Saint-Saëns
33077 Bordeaux
France

M.D. Cappellini
Istituto di Medicina Interna
Università degli Studi di Milano
Via Pace 9
20122 Milan
Italy

M. Charrel
Laboratoire de Chimie Biologique
Faculté de Médecine
27, Bd J. Moulin
13385 Marseille Cedex
France

U. Christians
Institut für Allgemeine Pharmakologie
Medizinische Hochschule Hannover
DW-3000 Hannover
Germany

M. Colledan
Centro Trapianto Fegato
Ospedale Maggiore IRCCS Milano
Istituto di Chirurgia Sperimentale
e dei Trapianti
Università degli Studi
Via F. Sforza 35
20122 Milan
Italy

A. Colombo
Centro Trapianto Fegato
Ospedale Maggiore
Policlinico di Milano
Università degli Studi di Milano
Via F. Sforza 35
20122 Milan
Italy

M. Colombo
Centro Trapianto Fegato
Ospedale Maggiore IRCCS Milano
Istituto di Chirurgia Sperimentale
e dei Trapianti
Università degli Studi
Via F. Sforza 35
20122 Milan
Italy

W. Concepcion
Pacific Transplant Institute
2340 Clay Street
San Francisco, CA 94115
USA

G. Covini
Institute of Internal Medicine
University of Milan
20122 Milan
Italy

P.J. Cozzone
Centre de Résonance Magnétique
Biologique et Médicale
27, Bd J. Moulin
13385 Marseille Cedex
France

R. D'Alba
Istituto di Scienze Biomediche
Via Donizetti 106
20052 Monza
Italy

C. Dalmasso
Laboratoire de Chimie Biologique
Faculté de Médecine
27, Bd J. Moulin
13385 Marseille Cedex
France

F. Desmoulin
Céntre de Résonance
Magnétique Biologique et Médicale
27, Bd J. Moulin
13385 Marseille Cedex
France

F. Dianzani
Institute of Virology
Viale di Porta Tiburtina, 28
00185 Rome
Italy

P. Di Mauro
Istituto di Anestesia e Rianimazione
dell'Università degli Studi
Ospedale Maggiore IRCCS Milano
Via F. Sforza 35
20122 Milan
Italy

M. D'Incalci
Istituto di Ricerche Farmacologiche
Mario Negri
Via Eritrea 62
20157 Milan
Italy

M. Doglia
Centro Trapianto Fegato
Ospedale Maggiore IRCCS Milano
Istituto di Chirurgia Sperimentale
e dei Trapianti
Università degli Studi
Via F. Sforza 35
20122 Milan
Italy

F. Donato
Centro Trapianto Fegato
Ospedale Maggiore IRCCS Milano
Istituto di Chirurgia Sperimentale
e dei Trapianti
Università degli Studi
Via F. Sforza 35
20122 Milan
Italy

M.G. Donelli
Istituto di Ricerche Farmacologiche
Mario Negri
Via Eritrea 62
20157 Milan
Italy

S.R. Dowd
Department of Biological Sciences
Carnegie Mellon University
Pittsburg, PA 15213
USA

C.O. Esquivel
Pacific Transplant Institute
2340 Clay Street
San Francisco, CA 94115
USA

S. Fargion
Istituto di Medicina Interna
Università di Milano
Via Pace, 9
20122 Milan
Italy

L.R. Fassati
Centro Trapianto Fegato
Ospedale Maggiore IRCCS Milano
Istituto di Chirurgia Sperimentale
e dei Trapianti
Università degli Studi
Via F. Sforza 35
20122 Milan
Italy

W. Feigl
Pathologisch-Bakteriologisches
Institut der Allgemeinen Poliklinik
A-1090 Vienna
Austria

G. Ferla
Centro Trapianto Fegato
Ospedale Maggiore IRCCS Milano
Istituto di Chirurgia Sperimentale
e dei Trapianti
Università degli Studi
Via F. Sforza 35
20122 Milan
Italy

G. Fiorelli
Istituto di Scienze Biomediche
Via Donizetti 106
20052 Monza
Italy

A.L. Fracanzani
Istituto di Scienze Biomediche
Via Donizetti 106
20052 Monza
Italy

J. Fung
Department of Surgery
University of Pittsburgh
School of Medicine
3601 Fifth Avenue
5c Falk Clinic
Pittsburgh, PA 15213
USA

J.-L. Gallis
Laboratoire de RMN de l'IBCN-CNRS
Université de Bordeaux II
1, rue Camille Saint-Saëns
33077 Bordeaux
France

D. Galmarini
Centro Trapianto Fegato
Ospedale Maggiore IRCCS Milano
Istituto di Chirurgia Sperimentale
e dei Trapianti
Università degli Studi
Via F. Sforza 35
20122 Milan
Italy

S. Gatti
Centro Trapianto Fegato
Ospedale Maggiore IRCCS Milano
Istituto di Chirurgia Sperimentale
e dei Trapianti
Università degli Studi
Via F. Sforza 35
20122 Milan
Italy

V. Gavazzeni
Istituto di Anestesia e Rianimazione dell'Università degli Studi
Ospedale Maggiore IRCCS Milano
Via F. Sforza 35
20122 Milan
Italy

D. Gentili
Istituto di Ricerche Farmacologiche Mario Negri
Via Eritrea 62
20157 Milan
Italy

C. Gettys
Pacific Transplant Institute
2340 Clay Street
San Francisco, CA 94115
USA

J.L. Gollan
Gastroenterology Division
Brigham and Women's Hospital
Harvard Medical School
Boston, MA 02115
USA

E. Gregnanin
Istituto di Anestesia e Rianimazione dell'Università degli Studi
Ospedale Maggiore IRCCS Milano
Via F. Sforza 35
20122 Milan
Italy

P.V. Grella
Institute of Gynecology and Obstetrics
University of Padua
Via Giustiniani, 3
35128 Padua
Italy

J. Grevel
Division of Immunology and Organ Transplantation and Division of Clinical Pharmacology
The University of Texas Medical School
6431 Fannin Street
Houston, TX 77030
USA

B. Gridelli
Centro Trapianto Fegato
Ospedale Maggiore IRCCS Milano
Istituto di Chirurgia Sperimentale e dei Trapianti
Università degli Studi
Via F. Sforza 35
20122 Milan
Italy

J-M. Gulian
Laboratoire de Chimie Biologique
Faculté de Médecine
27, Bd J. Moulin
13385 Marseille Cedex
France

H. Hartmann
Abteilung Gastroenterologie und Endokrinologie
Georg-August-Universität Göttingen
DW-3400 Göttingen
Germany

C. Ho
Department of Biological Sciences
Carnegie Mellon University
Pittsburgh, PA 15213
USA

P. Holzmüller
AG-NMR am Institut für Medizinische Physik
A-1090 Vienna
Austria

M. Johann
Service de Chirurgie Hépatobiliaire
Paul Brousse
94800 Villejuif
France

L. Kiffel
Inserm U75, CHU Necker
156 rue de Vaugirard
75015 Paris
France

S. Kusne
Department of Medicine, Infectious Disease and Surgery
University of Pittsburgh
School of Medicine
3601 Fifth Avenue
5c Falk Clinic
Pittsburgh, PA 15213
USA

M. Langer
Istituto di Anestesia e Rianimazione dell'Università degli Studi
Ospedale Maggiore IRCCS Milano
Via F. Sforza 35
20122 Milan
Italy

H.U. Lautz
Abteilung Gastroenterologie und Hepatologie
Medizinische Hochschule Hannover
DW-3000 Hannover 61
Germany

A. Lemoine
Inserm U75, CHU Necker
156 rue de Vaugirard
75015 Paris
France

G. Leonetti
Istituto di Clinica Medica Generale dell'Università degli Studi
Padiglione Sacco
Ospedale Maggiore IRCCS Milano
Via F. Sforza 35
20122 Milan
Italy

C.S. Lieber
Section of Liver Disease and Nutrition
Alcohol Research and Treatment Center
Bronx VA Medical Center and
Mt. Sinai School of Medicine
New York
USA

J. Lim
Pacific Transplant Institute
2340 Clay Street
San Francisco, CA 94115
USA

A. Lucianetti
Centro Trapianto Fegato
Ospedale Maggiore IRCCS Milano
Istituto di Chirurgia Sperimentale e dei Trapianti
Università degli Studi
Via F. Sforza 35
20122 Milan
Italy

U. Maggi
Centro Trapianto Fegato
Ospedale Maggiore IRCCS Milano
Istituto di Chirurgia Sperimentale e dei Trapianti
Università degli Studi
Via F. Sforza 35
20122 Milan
Italy

M. Martin
Department of Surgery
University of Pittsburgh
School of Medicine
3601 Fifth Avenue
5c Falk Clinic
Pittsburgh, PA 15213
USA

S. Masson
Centre de Résonance Magnétique Biologique et Médicale
27, Bd J. Moulin
13385 Marseille Cedex
France

E. Melada
Centro Trapianto Fegato
Ospedale Maggiore IRCCS Milano
Istituto di Chirurgia Sperimentale e dei Trapianti
Università degli Studi
Via F. Sforza 35
20122 Milan
Italy

E. Moser
AG-NMR am Institut für Medizinische Physik
A-1090 Vienna
Austria

R. Naccarato
Divisione di Gastroenterologia
Ospedale Monoblocco
Via Giustiniani 2
35128 Padua
Italy

P. Nakazato
Pacific Transplant Institute
2340 Clay Street
San Francisco, CA 94115
USA

M. Oellerich
Abteilung Klinische Chemie
Medizinische Hochschule Hannover
DW-3000 Hannover 61
Germany

P. Palazzi
Clinica Medica I
Università degli Studi di Milano
Via F. Sforza 35
20122 Milan
Italy

G. Paone
Centro Trapianto Fegato
Ospedale Maggiore IRCCS Milano
Istituto di Chirurgia Sperimentale e dei Trapianti
Università degli Studi
Via F. Sforza 35
20122 Milan
Italy

M. Parenti
Clinica Medica I
Università degli Studi di Milano
Via F. Sforza 35
20122 Milan
Italy

A. Piazzini
Centro Trapianto Fegato
Ospedale Maggiore IRCCS Milano
Istituto di Chirurgia Sperimentale e dei Trapianti
Università degli Studi
Via F. Sforza 35
20122 Milan
Italy

R. Pichlmayr
Klinik für Abdominal und Transplantationschirurgie
Medizinische Hochschule Hannover
DW-3000 Hannover 61
Germany

A. Piperno
Istituto di Scienze Biomediche
Via Donizetti 106
20052 Monza
Italy

A. Pollini
Istituto di Anestesia e Rianimazione dell'Università degli Studi
Ospedale Maggiore IRCCS Milano
Via F. Sforza 35
20122 Milan
Italy

G. Powis
Department of Pharmacology
Mayo Clinic and Foundation
200 First Street SW
Rochester, MN 55905
U.S.A.

P. Prato
Istituto di Anestesia e Rianimazione
Centro Trapianto di Fegato
Ospedale Maggiore
Policlinico di Milano
Università degli Studi di Milano
Via F. Sforza 35
20122 Milan
Italy

D. Proietti
Istituto di Anestesia e Rianimazione dell'Università degli Studi
Ospedale Maggiore IRCCS Milano
Via F. Sforza 35
20122 Milan
Italy

C. Reali Forster
Istituto di Anestesia e Rianimazione dell'Università degli Studi
Ospedale Maggiore IRCCS Milano
Via F. Sforza 35
20122 Milan
Italy

H. Reckendorfer
Pathologisch-Bakteriologisches
Institut der Allgemeinen Poliklinik
A-1090 Vienna
Austria

P. Reggiani
Centro Trapianto Fegato
Ospedale Maggiore IRCCS Milano
Istituto di Chirurgia Sperimentale e dei Trapianti
Università degli Studi
Via F. Sforza 35
20122 Milan
Italy

B. Ringe
Klinik für Abdominal und Transplantationschirurgie
Medizinische Hochschule Hannover
DW-3000 Hannover 61
Germany

R. Rivolta
Clinica Medica I
Università degli Studi di Milano
Via F. Sforza 35
20122 Milan
Italy

L. Rocchi
Istituto di Anestesia e Rianimazione dell'Università degli Studi
Ospedale Maggiore IRCCS Milano
Via F. Sforza 35
20122 Milan
Italy

R. Romano
Istituto di Scienze Biomediche
Via Donizetti 106
20052 Monza
Italy

R. Romito
Istituto di Anestesia e Rianimazione dell'Università degli Studi
Ospedale Maggiore IRCCS Milano
Via F. Sforza 35
20122 Milan
Italy

L. Rossaro
Divisione di Gastroenterologia
Ospedale Monoblocco
Via Giustiniani 2
35128 Padua
Italy

G. Rossi
Centro Trapianto Fegato
Ospedale Maggiore IRCCS Milano
Istituto di Chirurgia Sperimentale e dei Trapianti
Università degli Studi
Via F. Sforza 35
20122 Milan
Italy

M.G. Rumi
Institute of Internal Medicine
University of Milan
20122 Milan
Italy

D. Samuel
Service de Chirurgie Hépatobiliaire
Paul Brousse
94800 Villejuif
France

A. Sangiovanni
Institute of Internal Medicine
University of Milan
20122 Milan
Italy

V. Scantlebury
University of Pittsburgh
Department of Surgery
3601 Fifth Avenue
Falk Clinic 5 W
Pittsburgh, PA 15213
USA

C. Scheiner
Laboratoire d'Anatomie Pathologique
CHU Timone
27, Bd J. Moulin
13385 Marseille Cedex
France

H.M. Schiebel
Institut für Anorganische Chemie
TU Braunschweig
DW-3300 Braunschweig
Germany

F. Serino
Division of Immunology and Organ Transplantation and Division of Clinical Pharmacology
The University of Texas Medical School
6431 Fannin Street
Houston, TX 77030
USA

K.-Fr. Sewing
Institut für Allgemeine Pharmakologie
Medizinische Hochschule Hannover
DW-3000 Hannover
Germany

Sheila Sherlock
Royal Free Hospital
London NW3 2QG
UK

V. Simplaceanu
Department of Biological Sciences
Carnegie Mellon University
Pittsburgh, PA 15213
USA

M. Sperlich
Institut für Medizinische Physiologie
A-1090 Vienna
Austria

T.E. Starzl
Department of Surgery
University of Pittsburgh
School of Medicine
3601 Fifth Avenue
5c Falk Clinic
Pittsburgh, PA 15213
USA

R. Steininger
Chirurgische Universitätsklinik
University of Vienna
A-1090 Vienna
Austria

J.L. Szpakowski
Pacific Transplant Institute
2340 Clay Street
San Francisco, CA 94115
USA

D.H. Van Thiel
Department of Surgery
University of Pittsburgh
School of Medicine
3601 Fifth Avenue
Falk Clinic 5C
Pittsburgh, PA 15213
USA

R.P. Wood
Division of Immunology and Organ Transplantation and Division of Clinical Pharmacology
The University of Texas Medical School
6431 Fannin Street
Houston, TX 77030
USA

T. Wreghitt
Clinical Microbiology and
Public Health Laboratory
Addenbrooke's Hospital
Cambridge, CB2 2QW
UK

A. Zanchetti
Istituto di Clinica Medica
Generale e Terapia Medica
dell'Università degli Studi
Centro di Fisiologia Clinica e
Ipertensione
Ospedale Maggiore IRCCS Milano
Via F. Sforza 35
20122 Milan
Italy

M. Zucchetti
Istituto di Ricerche Farmacologiche
Mario Negri
Via Eritrea 62
20157 Milan
Italy

RISK ASSESSMENT IN LIVER TRANSPLANTATION FOCUS ON LUNG FUNCTION

Martin Langer, Eduardo Beck, Paolo Prato, Piero Di Mauro, Laura Rocchi, Chiara Reali Forster, Alberto Pollini, Emanuela Gregnanin, Daniela Proietti and Vittorio Gavazzeni

There is a general agreement that liver function, both preoperatively (including also the etiology of liver failure) and postoperatively, is the major determinant of the outcome in liver transplantation. Many organs are, however, involved in chronical liver disease and in the postoperative course of transplanted patients and these organs may fail even when the liver function is acceptable. Renal, hemodynamic and cardiac function, coagulation abnormalities have been extensively investigated in this context while lung function is less frequently addressed.

The interest in the respiratory function is obvious for anesthesiologists and intensivists, as providing respiratory support to assure adequate blood gases and tissue oxygenation is part of their specific responsibility.

Our relatively limited clinical experience with liver transplant patients at the liver transplant unit of the Ospedale Maggiore in Milan (136 liver transplants in 119 patients up to June 1991) does not allow to draw many conclusions but the aim of this contribution is to set the anesthesiologist's and intensivist's viewpoint. Figure 1 gives an overview on the problem "possible lung disfunction in liver transplant patients" which may arise at different times, before and after the operation.

D. Galmarini et al. (eds.), Drugs and the Liver: High Risk Patients and Transplantation, 1–9.

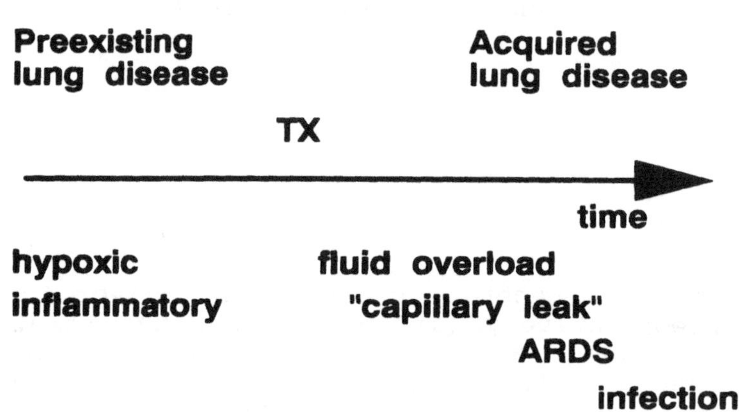

FIG. 1 - Occurrence of pulmonary complications in the liver transplant patient.

1.0 RISK FROM PREOPERATIVE LUNG DISFUNCTION

1.1 Hypoxia

Hypoxia is a very common finding in patients with end stage liver disease and may be mainly related to liver-associated abnormalities: intrapulmonary vascular dilatations or intrapulmonary shunt through arterio-venous channels (1,2) seem the most specific changes with a not yet well understood pathophysiology but with an increasing evidence of reversibility (3) if the patient overcomes the early post-transplant period. The investigations of Eriksson et al.(4) show that the arterial oxygen tension (PaO_2) could be correctly predicted from the multiple inert gas assessment of the ventilation/perfusion status of the lung. Even if this study cannot negate the presence of extrapulmonary right to left shunts (5), these shunts contribute only marginally to severe hypoxia in cirrhosis.

Hypoxic patients without evidence of parenchymal lung disease may have hypoxia from intrapulmonary vascular dilatations ("true shunt", only marginally responsive to airway pressure therapy or increased inspired oxygen fraction) or hypoxia from micro-atelectasis, pleural/peritoneal effusions or other causes of ventilation/perfusion mismatch (responsive to airway pressure therapy and increased inspired oxygen fraction). The different importance and the different risk coming from the same degree of hypoxia according to the underlying condition, both for the intraoperative and postoperative management, is evident and a careful evaluation of the oxygenation is an important part of the preoperative assessment. Different methods to investigate liver transplant candidates are proposed: the multiple inert gas elimination technique (6,4) is certainly the most complete and sofisticated method but it is also a rather complexe procedure and certainly not suitable for routine use. The easiest screening procedure in hypoxic patients is the evaluation of the arterial PO_2 after a short period of 100% oxygen breathing and the estimation of shunt by the use of a nomogram (7): a high inspired oxygen fraction increases the alveolar PO_2 even in lung units with very low ventilation-perfusion ratio (as atelectasis, for example) with a consequent consistent rise in arterial PO_2; however, if blood bypasses ventilated alveoli (intrapulmonary vascular dilatations - "true shunt") an high alveolar PO_2 will rise arterial PO_2 only slightly and just because of the additional dissolved O_2 from normally perfused and ventilated lung units. A true shunt>20%, estimated from the nomogram, should lead to further investigations, including pulmonary artery catheterization because of the possible association of clinically silent pulmonary hypertension. Figure 2 reports a flow chart for the evaluation of the hypoxic candidate to liver transplant.

1.2 Pretransplant lung inflammation

No data are available, to our knowledge, concerning the outcome of patients with chronic (COPD) or acute lung inflammation/bacterial infection before transplant.

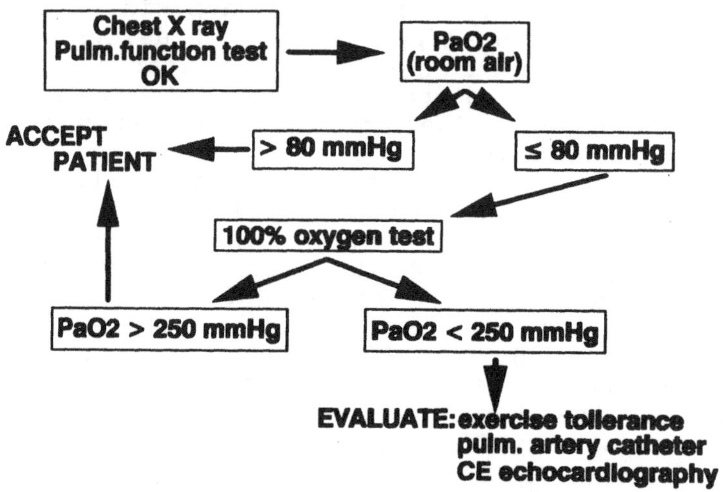

FIG. 2 - Hypoxia screening in the liver transplant candidate. Patients suspected to have a "true shunt">20% (see text) with $PaO_2 \leq 250$ mmHg when breathing 100% oxygen should have further investigations including contrast enhanced echocardiography, technetium 99 labeled macroaggregated albumin and extrapulmonary radionuclide scanning or multiple inert gas elimination, when available.

2.0 EARLY POSTOPERATIVE RESPIRATORY FAILURE

Also patients without overt preoperative hepatopulmonary syndrome frequently need prolonged postoperative respiratory support to assure adequate oxygenation.

2.1 Fluid overload

Preoperative fluid imbalance due to liver failure, massive intraoperative replacement and postoperative renal impairment lead easily to early postoperative fluid overload. In spite of the fact that each patient has his individual story, we performed a study to correlate early postoperative (until day 3) renal function (serum-creatinine) to cyclosporine-A (CyA) treatment (CyA blood levels), urinary output and central venous pressure (CVP) in 36 consecutive CyA treated patients. CyA was started intraoperatively as to reach and maintain blood levels of 800/900 ng/ml as soon as possible.

Data (Figure 3) were analyzed by analysis of variance and multiple regression analysis.

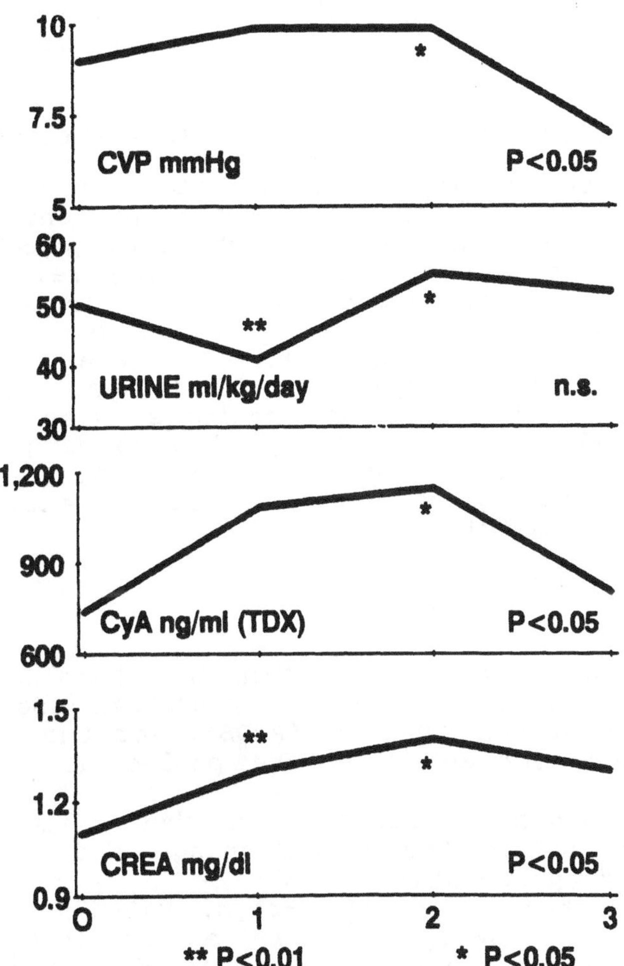

FIG. 3 - The variations over time and the interrelationship of serum creatinine, cyclosporine A polyclonal blood levels, urine output and central venous pressure during the first 3 postoperative days of 26 consecutive liver transplant recipients

The data show statistically significant variations of creatinine ($p<0.05$), CVP ($p<0.05$) and CyA ($p<0.05$) in the first 3 postoperative days and a correlation ($p<0.01$) for higher creatinine and lower urinary output at day 1 as well as a correlation ($p<0.05$) for higher creatinine, higher CyA level ($p<0.05$) and higher CVP ($p<0.05$) and lower urinary output ($p<0.05$) at day 2.

CyA nephrotoxicity frequently depresses urinary output, even when the intravascular volume is adequate; a low urinary output in these transplanted patients with a high turnover of fluids (fresh frozen plasma, parenteral nutrition, etc.) may lead to increasing filling pressures and consequently to a deterioration in lung function, requiring mechanical respiratory support.

2.2 Respiratory failure due to "capillary leak" or increased microvascular permeability

Like in gram negative sepsis, also during liver transplantation considerable amounts of endotoxins have been detected during the anhepatic phase (8). Endotoxin is well known to trigger the release of many mediators of inflammation, with an increase in vascular permeability and consequent fluid extravasation. In fact, the study of Miyata et al.(8) reports longer ventilator dependence and increased one-month case fatality in patients with higher levels of endotoxins. Obviously this finding is of great interest because of the current availability and proven efficacy of human monoclonal antibodies against endotoxin (9).

3.0 "ACQUIRED LUNG DISEASE" (ALD) AFTER LIVER TRANSPLANTATION

The most specific acquired pulmonary complications after liver transplantation are pneumonia and adult respiratory distress syndrome (ARDS). For the present purpose, pneumonia and ARDS are pooled as ALD and defined as:

"new and persistent infiltrate at chest film or CT scan, worsening of the gas exchange and positive microbiology" (pneumonia)

"diffuse opacities at chest X-rays, $PaO_2 \leq 75$ mmHg at $FiO_2 \geq 0.5$ with a severity score of at least 2.5, according to the scoring system proposed by Murray et al. (10)" (ARDS)

The importance of postoperative pulmonary complications (ALD) is well evident in Figure 4, where the survival is differentiated according to the occurence of ALD and to the subgroups "pneumonia without severe respiratory failure" and "ARDS", independently from the ethiology of this syndrome.

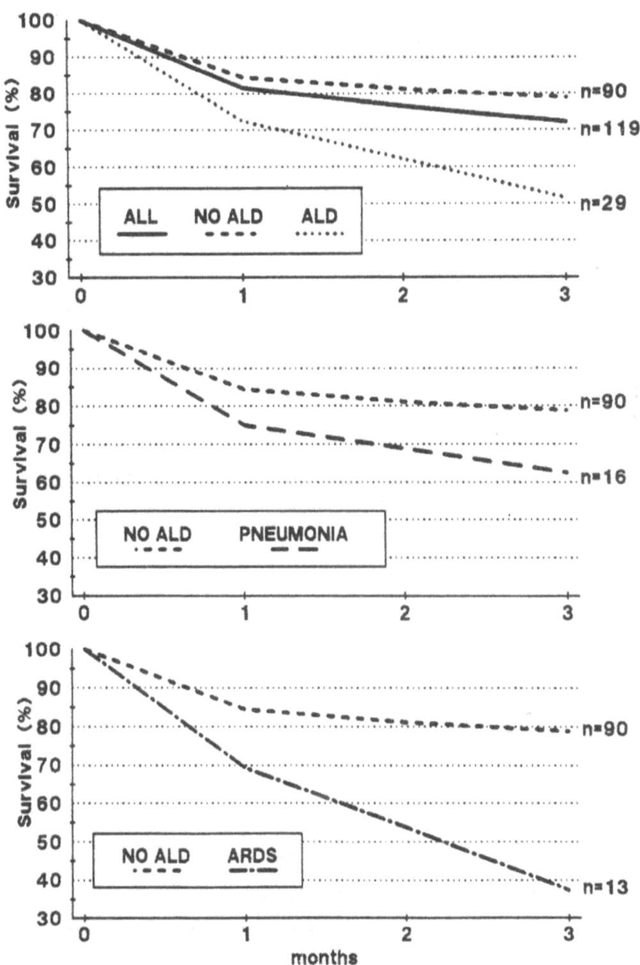

FIG. 4 - 3 months survival analysis of 119 patients (136 transplants) dividing the patients according the occurence of "ALD" (acquired lung disease = pneumonia and ARDS) or "No ALD" - upper part, "No ALD" or "pneumonia" - middle part, "No ALD" or "ARDS" - lower part (see text).

ARDS patients had the highest mortality, particularly when the respiratory failure was due to pulmonary and/or systemic infection (8/13 patients,

2 survivors). As the mortality rate is that high, an adequate risk assessment represents an important goal. We performed therefore a case control study considering the 8 overmentioned infective ARDS patients (cases) and 16 patients (controls) with similar pretransplant diagnosis and general conditions, treated in the same period by the same team. CMV donor/patient match, risk score (11), intraoperative blood loss, risk score on ICU admission (12), duration of ventilatory support, early graft function (assessed on day 3), renal function, other previous infection, graft rejection, treatment courses with monoclonal antibodies (OKT3), azathioprine, number of steroid boluses or steroid recyclings and mean CyA blood level before ARDS were investigated.

Our analysis was not able to define any of these parameters as a statistically significant risk factor for the development of ARDS after liver transplantation. The small number of cases is certainly the most obvious explanation for this unexpected result (a correlation between immunosuppressive treatment and infection is widely accepted); but also a multifactorial genesis seems to be involved in making the risk assessment of the most severe pulmonary complication rather difficult.

References

1. Krowka M.J., Tajik A.J., Dickson E.R., Wiesner R.H., Cortese D.A. (1990): Chest, 97: 1165-1170.

2. Sherlock S.(1988): Semin.Respir.Med., 9: 247-253.

3. Stoller J.K.(1990): Chest, 97: 1028-1030.

4. Eriksson L.S., Södermann C., Ericzon B.G., Eleborg L., Wahren J., Hedenstierna G.(1990): Hepatology, 12: 1350-1357.

5. Calabresi P., Abelmann W.H.(1957): J.Clin.Invest., 36: 1257-1265.

6. West J.B.(1977): In: Ventilation, Blood Flow and Gas Exchange, pp. 83-100. Blackwell Scientific Publications, Oxford.

7. West J.B.(1987): In: Pulmonary Pathophysiology - the essentials, pp. 172-187. Williams & Wilkins, Baltimore.

8. Miyata T., Todo S., Selby R., Yokoyama I., Tzakis A., Starzl T.E.(1989): Lancet, ii: 189-191.

9. Ziegler E.J., Fisher C.J., Sprung C.L., Straube R.C., Sadoff J.C., Foulke G.E., Wortel C.H., Fink M.P., Dellinger R.P.,

Teng N.N.H., Allen I.E., Berger H.J., Knatterud G.L., LoBuglio A.F., Smith C.R.and the HA-1A Sepsis Study Group (1991): N.Engl.J.Med., 324: 429-436.

10. Murray J.F., Matthay M.A., Luce J.M., Flick M.R.(1988): Am.Rev.Resp.Dis., 138: 720-723.

11. Shaw B.W., Wood R.P., Gordon R.D., Iwatsuki S., Gillquist W.P., Starzl T.E.(1985): Semin.Liver Dis., 5: 385-393.

12. Le Gall J., Loirat P., Alperovitch A., Glaser P., Grantil C., Mathieu D., Mercier P., Thomas R., Villers D. (1984): Crit. Care Med., 12: 975-977.

BIOCHEMICAL BASIS OF HEPATIC ISCHEMIC/REPERFUSION INJURY

Clifford A. Brass and John L. Gollan

INTRODUCTION

Based on observations in the intestine[1,2] heart[3,4] and kidney[5], as well as the liver[6], the concept of "reperfusion injury" has gained increasing attention in the transplant and organ preservation literature. This hypothesis proposes that there may be a separate distinct injury independent of the cellular injury which occurs during hypoxia or ischemia, associated with the resupply of blood (or oxygen) to previously ischemic (or hypoxic) mammalian tissue. Additionally, this reperfusion injury, under many circumstances, may be greater than the initial hypoxic insult. It has been postulated that the conversion of xanthine dehydrogenase (XDH) to the free radical producing enzyme, xanthine oxidase (XOD), during ischemia underlies this phenomenon. It is presumed that ATP breakdown[7] during the period of ischemia leads to the accumulation of the XOD substrate hypoxanthine, although the co-substrate, oxygen, is in limited supply. During reperfusion, oxygen is re-introduced and a burst of free radical production and cell injury ensues[8,9].

The above theory has gained widespread acceptance despite limited supportive data. The preponderance of data in support of this hypothesis is indirect and depends on the use of inhibitors of XOD activity (allopurinol) or free radical scavengers[10-12], which may have a variety of effects. Moreover, the few studies directly measuring XDH to XOD conversion in hypoxic

D. Galmarini et al. (eds.), Drugs and the Liver: High Risk Patients and Transplantation, 11–18.

tissues[13-15] have demonstrated a slow time course for this process that may be inconsistent with its purported role in mediating reperfusion injury. However, even more recent theories of reperfusion injury[16] (i.e. the no-reflow phenomenon) still implicate a burst of free radical production via xanthine oxidase (or some other as yet undefined mechanism) upon reoxygenation of previously ischemic tissue.

Because of the limited information available on the central biochemical changes underlying reperfusion injury, we have systematically examined the conversion of XDH to XOD during hypoxia. Our data demonstrates the conversion of XDH to XOD in a physiologically intact system (i.e. isolated perfused rat liver), and defines its relation to the duration and severity of hypoxia. We also document several physiological factors that modulate the temporal course of this conversion and may be highly relevant to the postulated role of XOD in underlying reperfusion injury.

METHODS

Isolated perfused rat liver (IPRL). Adult male Sprague-Dawley rats, either fed *ad libitum* (fed) or deprived of food for 16h (starved), were anesthetized, heparinized, and perfused through the portal vein with an oxygenated Krebs-Ringer bicarbonate buffer (KR). A recirculating perfusion system [17,18] containing 50ml of perfusate, included a membrane oxygenator, filter screen, bubble trap, pressure gauge, and temperature probe regulated at 37°C. Livers were perfused with a hemoglobin-free KR buffer, or with a perfluorochemical emulsion (Oxypherol, Alpha Therapeutics). Oxygen saturation was measured using a biological oxygen monitor, and bile was collected continuously via a bile duct cannula.

Experimental models. For global ischemia, the liver was placed in a beaker of unstirred Krebs medium at 37°C. To induce neutropenia, rats were exposed to 1,000 rads of whole body irradiation (Gamma Cell 40, Atomic Energy Canada) at a rate of 88 rads/min, ten days prior to study. In the "cardio-pulmonary arrest" (CPA) model of *in vivo* ischemia, a large incision was made in the diaphragm of an anesthetized rat. Complete cessation of respiratory movement and effective cardiac contraction occurred thereafter, and the surgical procedure to isolate the liver proceeded as usual 10 min after the initial incision into the diaphragm.

At the conclusion of each experiment, the liver was blotted dry and weighed, and a small wedge was resected from the right lobe of the liver and placed in 10% formalin and saline before sectioning and staining with hematoxylin and eosin. Additionally, where indicated, death was histologically quantified by a modification[17] of the trypan blue perfusion technique[19].

Xanthine oxidase/xanthine dehydrogenase assays. Liver samples were frozen in liquid nitrogen, pulverized and homogenized in a Polytron Homogenizer in a buffered solution (pH 7.8) containing 0.05 M potassium phosphate, 0.1 M EDTA, 0.5 mM dithiothreitol, and phenylmethyl-sulfonyl fluoride as described previously[17]. Where indicated, one half of the liver sample was homogenized without DTT so that the conformationally altered XDH molecule with xanthine oxidase activity (XODc) could be measured.

Homogenate was desalted in a G-25 column (Pharmacia) and assayed for XDH and XOD activity using a modification of the method of Waud and Rajagopalan[20], in the presence or absence of 6 mM NAD+ at 37°C. Aspartate aminotransferase and lactate dehydrogenase activities in the perfusate were measured spectrophotometrically using commercial kits (Sigma).

RESULTS

Studies with isolated perfused rat liver. Using a recirculating IPRL system, the liver from fed rats was perfused with oxygenated Krebs buffer for 30 min, followed by hypoxic perfusion for an additional 180 min. XOD activity increased from 25-45% during this period with a close correlation between the duration of hypoxia and XOD activity (Fig. 1; r=0.97). Enzyme conversion was inversely related to the level of oxygen consumption at 2.5h (Fig. 2; r=0.92). These changes occurred in a functionally intact system, as assessed by resumption of oxygen consumption (1.75 Nmol O_2/min/g) and bile flow (3 Nl/min) upon reoxygenation after 2h of hypoxia in this system. Additionally, hepatocellular injury as assessed by both AST and LDH release as well as cell death measured by trypan blue uptake (3%) were extremely low.

Factors influencing xanthine dehydrogenase to xanthine oxidase conversion. A model of global ischemia was employed to investigate factors that may modulate the conversion of hepatic XDH to XOD. There was a gradual increase in percent XOD activity in the liver of fed animals over the 2.5h period of anoxia, however, this conversion was accelerated in the livers from fasted animals (Fig. 3). In our cardio-pulmonary arrest model simulating *in vivo* ischemia, there was no significant change in conversion to XOD activity in the livers of fed animals. However, there was a dramatic increase in hepatic XOD activity in animals subjected to cardio-pulmonary arrest (n=32), relative to fasted controls (n=17: Fig. 3). This effect was seen only after a period of hypoxia, but was significant as early as 30 min into the anoxic period. This intervention also led to significantly greater hepatic edema ($p<0.05$) with an increase in water content in the liver after anoxia in the starved/CPA group (51±4%) almost twice that noted in the livers of fed (24±3%), fed/CPA (29±4%), or starved (20±4%) animals. This was accompanied by extensive vacuolization of hepatocytes as well as eosinophilic degeneration in the starved/CPA group alone. No zonal differences in the pattern of injury were noted.

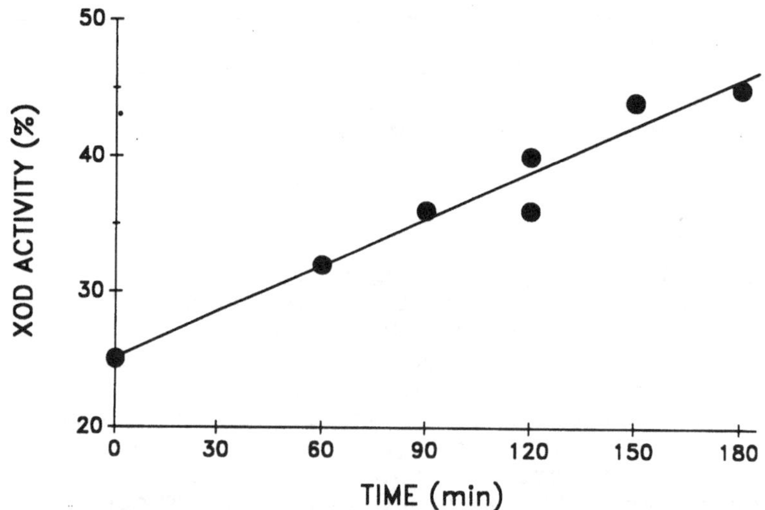

Figure 1. Conversion to xanthine oxidase activity (% XOD) during hypoxia in IPRL. Each point represents the % XOD activity [XOD/(XOD + XDH)] measured at the end of the perfusion period (r=0.97).

It has been postulated that XODc (DTT-labile XOD) may be the major intermediate for cleavage to XODe[14]. In our studies of anoxic liver, DTT-labile XOD activity increased after 90 min of ischemia (anoxia) only in the livers of the starved/CPA group (18±2% vs. 0-2±1%). This activity was not present at 0 min, but increased progressively over a 2h period of anoxia. In assessing total XOD activity, after 90 min of ischemia, 75% of the total XDH plus XOD activity was in the XOD form. By 2h, conversion to XOD activity (90%) was virtually complete in this group.

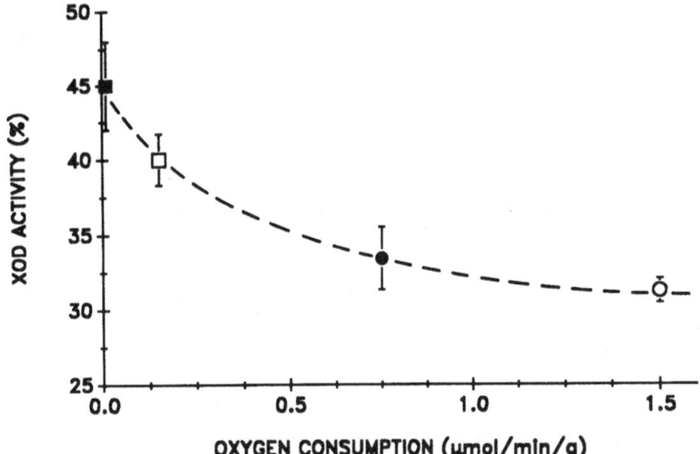

Figure 2. Conversion to xanthine oxidase activity as a function of hepatic oxygen consumption. Livers from fed rats were exposed to different levels of oxygenation by perfusion with oxygenated Oxypherol (○), oxygenated Krebs-bicarbonate buffer (•), nitrogen-saturated Krebs buffer (□), or incubation in Krebs buffer (■) without perfusion for 150 min. Each point represents the mean±SE of the % XOD conversion in 6 or more perfused livers (r=0.92).

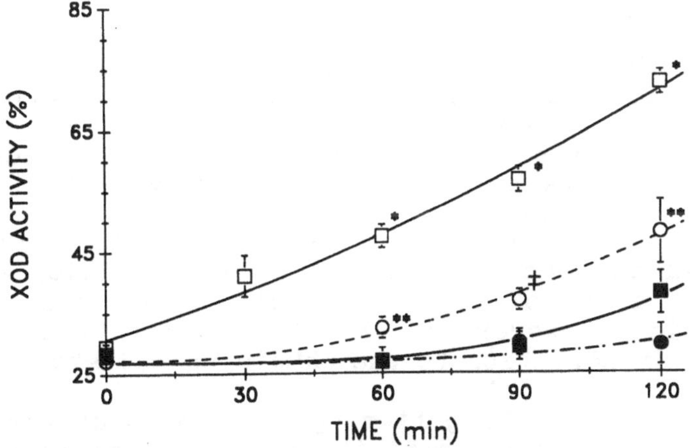

*Figure 3. Conversion of xanthine dehydrogenase to XOD activity during ischemia. Each point represents the mean±SE of at least 3 rat livers (n=76). Livers were obtained from rats fed ad libitum (•-•-•) or fasted for 16 h (○--○). Cardiopulmonary arrest (■—■) involved cutting the diaphragm of the anesthetized rat and delaying completion of surgical removal of the liver for a 10-min period of in vivo ischemia. The effect of this intervention in fasted animals is denoted by (□—□). *P < 0.01 vs. starved or fed/cardiopulmonary arrest; **P < 0.01 vs. fed; ‡P < vs. fed.*

Potential mechanisms of the cardio-pulmonary arrest effect. Thrombosis did not appear to be the mechanism of the CPA effect in that pre-heparinization of animals had no effect on the rate of formation of XOD activity (70±4%, n=6) in the liver of starved/CPA rats, compared to non-heparinized animals (73±4%, n=6), after 2.5h of ischemia. In addition, circulating white cells did not appear to play a role in this CPA effect since there was no difference noted in conversion to percent XOD after 90 min of global ischemia when neutropenic animals (52±5%) or non-neutropenic animals (57±2%) were studied.

DISCUSSION

These data demonstrate conversion to the free radical-producing state (increased XOD activity) in functional liver, as reflected by continued oxygen utilization and bile production after reoxygenation, as a function of both the degree and duration of hypoxia. Although these findings confirm the long held, but previously undemonstrated, tenets of the xanthine oxidase theory of reperfusion injury[7,9], the relatively slow conversion to XOD activity (25-45% XOD over a 3h period) raises the question of the physiological relevance of this enzymatic conversion. To address this issue, we investigated several variables that may modulate and potentially enhance this response to hypoxia.

The literature contains conflicting reports on the effects of nutritional status on ischemic and reperfusion injury[21-24]. In our model of global ischemia, overnight fasting clearly led to an increased conversion to xanthine oxidase activity. This may be due to any number of changes that accompany an overnight fast including depletion of glycogen[25], decreased glutathione levels[24], and alteration of the hormonal milieu of the liver. The importance of this observation, however, is that it now shifts the focus in organ preservation to the physiological state of the organ donor.

Our most striking finding, the rapid acceleration and conversion to XOD activity in starved animals after a brief period of *in vivo* hypoxia (cardio-pulmonary arrest), remains without a precise explanation. In light of growing data implicating neutrophil-endothelial cell adhesion as underlying ischemia/reperfusion injury, we repeated these experiments in neutrophil depleted animals. Our data demonstrates no role for white cells in mediating the effects produced in the cardio-pulmonary arrest model.

Finally, these effects did not appear to be an artifact secondary to thrombosis within the liver.

Although our data clearly define changes in XOD activity, and the physiological modulation of such changes, that are consistent with both the older hypothesis of reperfusion injury[7-9], as well as the more recent "no-reflow" theories of reperfusion injury[4,26], these studies do not definitively answer the question of the causality of increased XOD activity mediating *subsequent* reperfusion damage. We noted an association of marked histologic injury in the group with the maximal increase in XOD activity (starved/CPA group), and there is some data suggesting that the increase in xanthine oxidase is merely a reflection of cellular injury[27]. However, our observations of significant increases in XOD conversion unaccompanied by any detectable edema or histologic changes, or any significant cell death as assessed by AST release or trypan blue uptake, tend to contradict this notion. More importantly, the increased activity of XODc (DTT-labile XOD, the conformationally altered XDH molecule with XOD activity) is likely attributable to alterations in the redox state in the anoxic cells[28] (reflecting oxidation of several of the 14 sulfhydryl groups in the XDH molecule to disulfides) indicative of altered cell physiology during hypoxia rather than cell death with concomitant protease release. This view is consistent with other data suggesting that it is this altered XDH molecule (XODc) that precedes enzymatic cleavage to the smaller XOD molecule[14].

Collectively, our findings present important evidence that conversion to XOD activity may occur in a functionally intact liver and, under certain conditions, within a time course consistent with its purported physiological role in mediating reperfusion injury. However, a more definitive demonstration of the role of XOD in reperfusion injury awaits further development of sophisticated methods to study individual cells, as well as determination of the role of XOD within different cell types within the liver (i.e. hepatocytes, endothelial cells, Kupffer cells). Of direct clinical relevance, however, these findings suggest that the pre-morbid condition of organ donors, specifically the nutritional status and the ischemic/ hypoxic state, may be important factors in achieving optimal organ storage and minimizing hepatocellular injury.

REFERENCES

1. Parks D.A., Bulkley G.B. and Granger D.N. (1983):*Surgery*, 94:428-433.
2. Parks D.A. and Granger D.N. (1986):*Am. J. Physiol.*, 250: G749-G753.
3. Schaper J., and Schaper W. (1983):*J. Am. Coll. Cardiol.*, 1:1037-1046.
4. Simpson P.J., Mickelson J.K. and Lucchesi B.R. (1987):*Fed. Proc.*, 46:2413-2421.
5. Owens M.L., Harrison M.L., Wolcott M.W., Maxwell J.G. and Taylor J.B. (1974):*Transplantation*, 17:424-427.
6. Thurman R.G., Marzi I., Seitz G., Thies J., LeMasters J.J. and Zimmerman F. (1988):*Transplantation*, 46:502-506.
7. Roy R.S. and McCord J.M. (1983): In: *Oxy radicals and their scavenger systems*. Vol. II., edited by R.A. Greenwald and G. Cohen, pp. 145-153. Elsevier/North Holland. Amsterdam.
8. Adkison D., Hollwarth M.E., Benoit J.N., Parks D.A., McCord J.M., and Granger D.N. (1986) *Acta. Physiol. Scand.*, Suppl. 548:101-107.
9. McCord J.M. (1985):*N. Engl. J. Med.* 312:159-163.
10. Nordstrom G., Seeman T., and Hasselgren P.O. (1985):*Surgery*, 97:679-683.
11. Atalla S.L., Toledo-Pereyra L.H., MacKenzie G.H. and Cederna J.P. (1985):*Transplantation*, 40:584-589.
12. Marubayashi S., Dohi K., Ochi K., and Kawasaki T. (1986):*Surgery*, 90:184-191.
13. Engerson T.D., McKelvey T.G., Rhyne D.B., Boggio E.B., Snyder S.J., and Jones H.P. (1986):*J. Clin. Invest.*, 79:1564-1570.
14. McKelvey T.G., Hollwarth M.E., Granger D.N., Engerson T.D., Landler U. and Jones H.P. (1988):*Am. J. Physiol.*, 254:G753-G760.
15. Parks D.A., Williams T.K. and Beckman J.S. (1988):*Am. J. Physiol.*, 25:G768-G774.
16. Schmid-Schoenbein G.W. and Engler R.L. (1988): *Microvascular Res.*, 23:273.
17. Brass C.A., Narciso J. and Gollan J.L. (1991): *J. Clin. Invest.*, 87:424-431.
18. Gollan J.L., Hammaker L., Licko V., and Schmid R. (1981):*J. Clin. Invest.*, 67:1003-1015.
19. Belinsky S.A., Popp J.A., Kauffman F.C. and Thurman R.G. (1984):*J. Pharmacol. Exp. Ther.*, 230:755-760, 1984.
20. Waud W.R. and Rajagopalan K.V. (1976):*Arch. Biochem. Biophys.*, 172:354-356.
21. Jennische, E. (1983):*Acta Physiol. Scand.*, 118:69-73.
22. Anundi I. and DeGroot H. (1989):*Am. J. Physiol.*, 25:G58-G64.
23. Bradford B.U., Marotto M., LeMasters J.J. and Thurman R.G. (1986):*J. Pharm. Exper. Ther.*, 236:263-268.
24. Younes M. and Strubelt O. (1988):*Res. Commun. Chem. Path. Pharm.* 59:369-381.
25. Jennische E. (1984):*Acta. Path. Microbiol. Immunol. Scand.*, 92:55-64.
26. Engler R.G., Dahlgren M.D., Morris D.D., Peterson M.A. and Schmid-Schonbein G.W. (1986):*Am. J. Physiol.*,251:H314-H322.
27. DeGroot H. and Littauer A. (1989):*Free Radical Biol. Med.*, 6:541-551.
28. Waud W.R and Rajagopalan K.V. (1976):*Arch. Biochem. Biophys.*, 172:365-379.

DONOR RATING AND ASSESSMENT OF PRETRANSPLANT PROGNOSIS BY USE OF THE MEGX TEST

M.Oellerich , M.Burdelski , H.U.Lautz , H.Hartmann , B.Ringe , R.Pichlmayr

INTRODUCTION

It is well recognized that liver disease or dysfunction may influence the disposition of drugs. Conversely, it has been suggested to use the hepatic drug metabolising capacity as a measure of liver function (1). Recently, a test has been described (2) which is based on the cytochrome P-450-mediated formation of the lidocaine metabolite monoethylglycinexylidide (MEGX). This test is rapid and easy to perform. A loss of hepatic cytochrome P-450 activity or major changes of hepatic blood flow, for instance due to portosystemic shunting, result in a decrease of MEGX formation.
Figure 1 shows MEGX formation kinetics after an intravenous bolus of lidocaine injected (1 mg/kg) over about two minutes. The highest MEGX test results were observed in liver donors with unimpaired organ function and in normal subjects. Liver recipients with uncomplicated postoperative course showed somewhat lower test results on postoperative day 28. In patients with cirrhosis the increase of MEGX concentration in serum was much less expressed and dependent on disease severity. No MEGX formation was detectable after complete removal of the liver in a recipient during the unhepatic phase of transplantation. This finding suggests that potential sources of extrahepatic MEGX formation have no noticeable

D. Galmarini et al. (eds.), Drugs and the Liver: High Risk Patients and Transplantation, 19–24.

influence on the MEGX test.

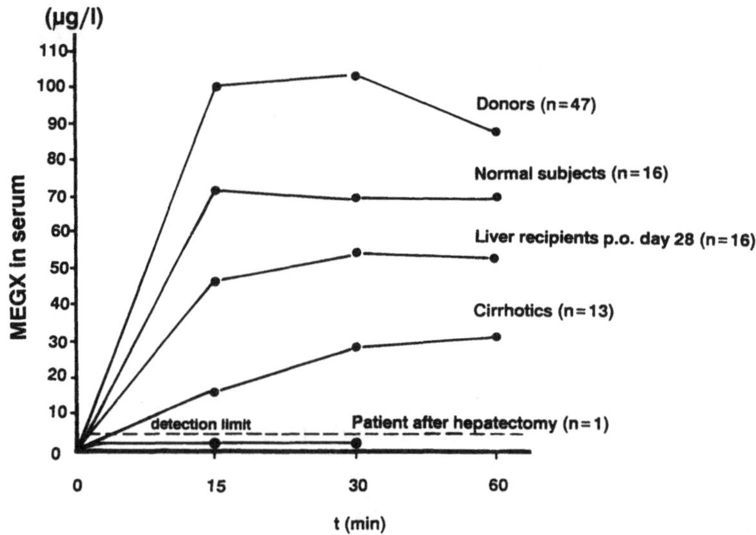

Fig. 1. Serum concentration-time curves of MEGX.

DONOR LIVER QUALITY ASSESSMENT

The improvement of donor selection criteria is important to achieve optimum utilization of the limited donor pool. Data from a recent prospective study with 171 donor/recipient pairs indicate that the functional state of the donor liver as assessed by lidocaine metabolite formation plays an important role for the early outcome of transplantation (3). The probability of graft survival for 120 days was significantly higher for livers from donors with MEGX test results above 90 µg/l ($p=0.0001$). The percentage of patients with liver tumors, cirrhosis, and graft failure was comparable in the groups with MEGX values > 90 µg/l or ≤ 90 µg/l. The lowest probability of graft survival was found for livers from donors with MEGX values less than 50 µg/l. About two-thirds of grafts from donors with MEGX values ≤ 50 µg/l survived less than 20 days the most frequent cause of graft loss being primary graft nonfunction.

From postoperative day 20 to day 119, septicaemia was the major cause of death independent from MEGX test results.

In not-used donors MEGX test results showed a large variation. The data from two recent studies with not-accepted donors indicate that at least 36% (3) or 60% (4) of organs not used might have been suitable for transplantation according to MEGX test results above 90 µg/l and 100 µg/l respectively.

Previous investigations have shown that moderate or severe steatosis of the donor liver may carry a substantial risk regarding the early outcome of transplantation (5). So far, only few data are available on MEGX formation in steatotic liver grafts (6). Grafts with mild steatosis showed predominantly favorable MEGX test results and functioned as well as normal grafts. In two cases with moderate steatosis (ca. 50%) decreased MEGX test results were observed which ranged from < 3 to 41 µg/l. Such livers may be more susceptible to early postoperative complications. However, the few observations do not allow final conclusions about the suitability of steatotic donor livers.

In a recent study (3) a stepwise survival analysis was performed by use of the Cox proportional hazards model using data from 51 donor/recipient pairs. It could be demonstrated that none of the evaluated conventional tests contributed to a further improvement of our predictive ability when added to the values of MEGX and the histological findings. These results confirm that in contrast to the MEGX test, current methods of donor assessment are highly inefficient at predicting early graft function.

Determination of MEGX formation in donors and in the corresponding transplant recipients on the first postoperative day revealed a substantial decrease of test results (mean: 49%) over this interval (3). This finding seems to reflect a drop of the oxidative metabolising capacity of the graft, presumably due to harvesting, preservation, and reperfusion damage. These factors and the recipient status also influence early graft survival. It is therefore not surprising that in some cases graft loss occurred despite favorable donor MEGX test results. In most cases with primary graft nonfunction, low MEGX test results were observed in donors and in the corresponding recipients. Decreased MEGX values have been found in rare cases with episodes of severe arterial hypotension or after administration of a wrong test dose.

Based on current experience it is suggested to interpret MEGX test results with regard to donor liver quality assessment as follows: less than 50 µg/l (bad), 50-90 µg/l (questionable), and greater than 90 µg/l (good). The results of the MEGX test should be used for donor organ classification in combination with generally accepted features of clinical assessment (6). Currently available data suggest that the MEGX test is a valuable tool for the selection of donor organs.

ASSESSMENT OF PRETRANSPLANT PROGNOSIS

The availability of appropriate predictors of pretransplant survival would be helpful to improve selection criteria for transplant candidates and thus the timing of transplantation.

In a recent prospective study we have examined the prognostic value of the flow-dependent MEGX and ICG tests, the Pugh score, and traditional biochemical liver function tests in adult patients with advanced cirrhosis (7). Patients who underwent orthotopic liver transplantation within the follow-up period of 365 days were excluded. 101 patients with biopsy proven cirrhosis were studied. During the follow-up period 28 patients died of their liver diseases. At entry we recorded indocyanine green (ICG) half-life, MEGX formation, bilirubin (BIL) and albumin (ALB) serum concentrations, activities of cholinesterase (CHE) and alkaline phosphatase (AP), prothrombin time (PT), the presence of ascites (ASC) and encephalopathy (ENC), and in addition the Pugh score. These variables were subjected as covariates to a stepwise survival analysis by use of the Cox proportional hazards model. At the final step Pugh score, MEGX formation, and ICG half-life were found to be the only independent variables significantly related to one-year survival. None of the parameters evaluated contributed to a further improvement of our predictive ability when added to the values of the Pugh score (improvement: $p<0.0005$), MEGX (improvement: $p=0.005$), and ICG (improvement: $p=0.072$). As single parameters MEGX, ICG, and Pugh score showed only a moderate prognostic sensitivity (54-61%). Therefore, we investigated whether an appropriate combination of these statistically independent tests would increase sensitivity. The parallel combination of Pugh score and MEGX test yielded a substantially higher prognostic sensitivity (82%).

These findings suggest that an improved index of hepatic function could be developed by combining the Pugh score with one of the studied flow-dependent dynamic liver function tests. In clinical practice MEGX formation appears to be the flow-dependent test of choice as it is universally available and easy to perform.

Based on these considerations, we have developed a modification of the Pugh score. Using the grading system described by Pugh et al. (8) one, two, or three points are scored for increased abnormality

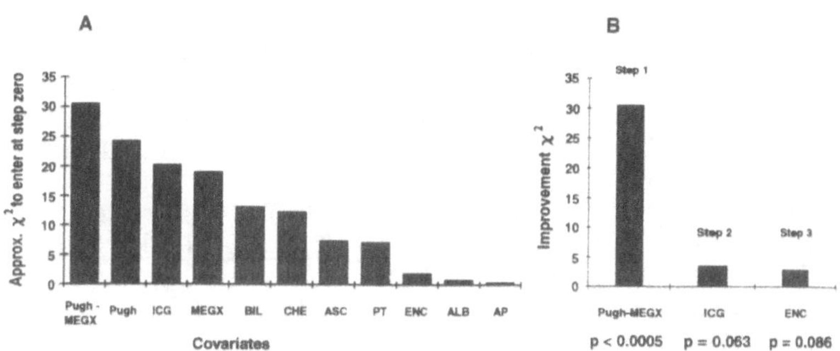

Fig. 2. Significant predictors of one-year survival in cirrhotics. A: Influence of transplant candidate variables as covariates on the hazard function in the Cox model. B: Summary of stepwise results.

of MEGX test results (MEGX > 30 µg/l: one point; 10-30 µg/l: two points; < 10 µg/l: three points). For each patient of our study (7) the modified Pugh-MEGX score was calculated by adding the points obtained from the MEGX test to those of the original Pugh score. This novel Pugh-MEGX score and the remaining variables including the original Pugh score were again subjected as covariates to a stepwise survival analysis by use of the Cox model.

The data from the Cox regression analysis suggest that out of the parameters studied, the Pugh-MEGX score was the best indicator of one-year survival in this population of transplant candidates (Fig. 2). The resulting improvement of our predictive ability was very small when ICG test results and data on the presence or absence of encephalopathy were added to the Pugh-MEGX score. A prospective study is in progress to investigate the prognostic value of the Pugh-MEGX score in patients with chronic liver disease.

In conclusion, the MEGX test appears to be a promising approach for the assessment of pretransplant prognosis in patients with advanced cirrhosis.

REFERENCES

1. Branch R.A. (1982): *Hepatology*, 2: 97-105.
2. Oellerich M., Burdelski M., Ringe B., Lamesch P., Gubernatis G., Bunzendahl H., Pichlmayr R., Herrmann H. (1989): *Lancet*, 1: 640-642.
3. Oellerich M., Burdelski M., Ringe B., Wittekind Ch., Lamesch P., Lautz H.U., Gubernatis G., Beyrau R., Pichlmayr R. (1991): *Transplant. Proc.*, 23: 1575-1578.
4. Schroeder T.J., Pesce A.J., Ryckman F.C., Brunson M.E., Tresler T.B., Pedersen S.H., Tchervenkov J.I., Penn I., Alexander J.W., Balistreri W.F. (1991): *Ann. Clin. Sci.*, in press.
5. Todo S., Demetris A.J., Makowka L., Teperman L., Podesta L., Shaver T., Tzakis A., Starzl T.E. (1989): Transplantation, 47: 903-905.
6. Oellerich M., Burdelski M., Ringe B., Ozaki N., Binder L., Pichlmayr R. (1991): In: *Therapy in Liver Disease*, edited by J. Rodes and V. Arroyo Ediciones Doyma, S.A., Barcelona, in press.
7. Oellerich M., Burdelski M., Lautz H.U., Binder L., Pichlmayr R. (1991): *Hepatology*, 14: in press.
8. Pugh R.N.H., Murray-Lyon I.M., Dawson J.L., Pietroni M.C., Williams R. (1973): *Br. J. Surg.*, 60: 646-649.

SIGNIFICANCE OF CYCLOSPORINE PHARMACOKINETICS IN LIVER TRANSPLANTATION

J. Grevel, R.P. Wood, and F. Serino

Pharmacokinetics is the science of the biological processes from drug administration to drug elimination. These processes can best be followed as the changes in drug concentration in biological fluids such as blood. Cyclosporine pharmacokinetics are characterized by a large intersubject variability (1). Pharmacodynamics is the science of the interactions between drug concentrations in the body and drug effects. The pharmacodynamics of cyclosporine show therapeutic and toxic concentrations in close proximity, i.e., the therapeutic range of cyclosporine concentration is narrow (2). This situation is further complicated in liver transplantation where the transplanted organ plays a key role in the pharmacokinetics of cyclosporine.

PHARMACOKINETICS

Cyclosporine absorption after oral dosing is incomplete and dependent upon the availability of bile in the small intestine (3). The bioavailability of cyclosporine ranges between 20 and 40% during periods of normal graft function. In the absence of bile, such as during bile drainage through a T-tube, the bioavailability is erratic and frequently as low as 5% (4). For that reason, cyclosporine is administered intravenously for the first days after liver transplantation until the patient can tolerate solid food. Indeed, it has been demonstrated that food which triggers bile flow enhances cyclosporine absorption (5). The fraction of the oral dose which reaches the central circulation intact (bioavailability) is not determined by the first pass effect of the liver, but rather by the

D. Galmarini et al. (eds.), Drugs and the Liver: High Risk Patients and Transplantation, 25–30.

absorption from the upper part of the small intestine into the portal blood stream (3).

Around 40% of cyclosporine in whole blood is associated with red blood cells. This percentage is lower in patients with abnormally low hematocrits (6). In plasma, only 4 to 12% of cyclosporine are not bound to proteins (7). Most plasma binding involves lipoproteins: 10% to VLDL, 30% to LDL, and 40% to HDL (8). Lipoprotein-bound cyclosporine is likely to be pharmacologically active in vivo since both lymphocytes (the therapeutic targets) and hepatocytes (the site of metabolism) carry LDL receptors in the cell membrane (9). Furthermore, cyclosporine packaged into lipsomes was more potent than free cyclosporine in an in vitro lymphocyte proliferation assay (10).

Many of the problems of immunosuppression based on cyclosporine in liver transplant patients are derived from the fact that the transplanted organ is the main site of cyclosporine elimination. In the case of cyclosporine, systemic clearance and hepatic clearance are identical. Unchanged cyclosporine is neither eliminated in urine nor in bile (11). Metabolites, however, appear in high concentrations in bile, and they undergo enterohepatic recycling (11). During impaired bile drainage as indicated by increases in serum bilirubin, metabolite concentrations in blood can rise dramatically (11) together with concentration measurements by nonspecific assays. Assuming that metabolites of cyclosporine are not pharmacologically active, only specific assay methods were recommended for the monitoring of liver transplant patients (12).

PHARMACODYNAMICS

In vitro, it was shown that all known metabolites are weaker immunosuppressive agents than cyclosporine itself (13). More recently, however, Kunzendorf et al. reported significant differences in nonspecific cyclosporine measurements in serum between rejecting and nonrejecting renal transplant patients (14). In whole blood, these differences could not be demonstrated when a specific assay for unchanged cyclosporine was used. There is basically only one explanation for these findings, i.e., cyclosporine metabolites are involved in the prevention of rejection. This conclusion was independently confirmed in another group of renal transplant patients (15). Furthermore, the main cyclosporine metabolite in humans was related to central nervous system toxicity in a renal transplant patient (16). Unfortunately, there are no convincing animal or in vitro models to test the toxicity of cyclosporine metabolites.

The therapeutic effects of cyclosporine and its metabolites cannot be measured as graded responses in transplant patients. The quantal nature of the responses is defined as the absence or presence of rejection episodes. In Table 1, steady state concentrations (Css) determined by the AVC method (17) and trough levels (TL) measured by a nonspecific fluorescence polarization immunoassay in serum (TDX) and by a liquid chromatographic method in whole blood (LC) are compared between rejecting and nonrejecting renal transplant patients (15).

TABLE 1. Correlation of Css and TL with renal graft rejection

Assay	TDX				LC			
Concen-tration	CSS		TL		CSS		TL	
Rejection	N	Y	N	Y	N	Y	N	Y
Mean or median (ng/ml)	156	120	68	65	268	242	104	99
Signifi-cance level	0.06[a]		0.86[b]		0.44[a]		0.78[b]	

Table 1 shows that the Css concentration as determined by the TDX assay in serum reached an average nadir of 156 ng/ml in patients without rejection during the first 40 days after transplantation. Patients who rejected had their Css drop significantly lower. These differences were not seen with TL nor with any concentration measured by LC.

INDIVIDUALIZATION OF CYCLOSPORINE THERAPY

The large intersubject variability of cyclosporine clearance renders any standard dosing regimen either ineffective or dangerous. According to the Wilkinson and Shand model of hepatic drug clearance (18), cyclosporine clearance should be independent of hepatic blood flow, but dependent upon changes in the intrinsic activity of the metabolizing enzymes (cytochrome P450). Hepatic dysfunction as evidenced by an increase in serum bilirubin concentrations was correlated with a reduced cyclosporine clearance in bone marrow transplant patients (19) and in renal transplant patients (20). Cyclosporine clearance corrected for body size decreased with increasing age between 1 month and adulthood (21). Age and liver function are by far the most important demographic factors which determine cyclosporine clearance.

Drug interactions account for both interindividual and intraindividual variability in cyclosporine pharmacokinetics. Table 2 categorizes well-documented interactions (22).

TABLE 2. Drug interactions

Cyclosporine concentrations increase	Cyclosporine concentrations decrease	Nephrotoxicity increases
aminoglycoside antibiotics	carbamazepin	aminoglycoside antibiotics
diltiazem	isoniazid	amphotericin B
ketoceonazol (and related compounds)	phenobarbital	
steroids (high doses)	phenytoin	cimitidine
Metoclopramide	rifampin	contrimoxazole
nicardipine		macrolide antibiotics
verapamil		

Certain drug interactions can be exploited to the benefit of the patient. The calcium channel blockers diltiazem (23) and verapamil (24) have been proposed as standard concomitant medications to increase cyclosporine concentrations and to simultaneously protect the patient from the increased risk of nephrotoxicity.

Liver transplant patients may benefit like renal transplant patients (25) from individual cyclosporine doses right from the start. While in this case parmacokinetic studies before liver transplantation are useless, it is still possible to obtain an estimate of the clearance of cyclosporine shortly after anastomosis of the graft. A short term cyclosporine infusion produces measurable cyclosporine concentrations in the central circulation. Concentrations are determined in the portal vein (C_{PV}) and the hepatic vein (C_{HV}), and the hepatic extraction ration (E) of cyclosporine can be calculated as follows:

$$E = \frac{C_{PV} - C_{HV}}{C_{PV}}$$

For this estimate of E, the potential difference in concentration between portal vein and hepatic artery can be neglected. By further estimating the hepatic blood flow (Q) from the patients' size and age, one can calculate his/her individual cyclosporine clearance:

$$CL = Q \times E$$

Knowing the clearance and the therapeutic target steady state concentration, the individual infusion rate (IR) of cyclosporine can be calculated:

$$IR = CL \times Css$$

Experiments are presently underway to prove the usefulness of this design.

REFERENCES

1. Ptachcinski R.J., Venkataramanan R. and Burkart G.J., (1986): Clin. Pharmacokin. 11: 107-132.
2. Kahan B.D., Wideman C.A., Ried M., Gibbons S., Jarowenko M., Flechner S. and Van Buren C.T., (1984): Transplant. Proc. 16: 1195-1199.
3. Grevel J., (1986): Transplant. Proc. 18 (Suppl.5): 9-15.
4. Tredger J.M., Grevel J., Naoumov N., Steward C.M., Niven A.A., Whiting B. and Williams R., (1991): Eur. J. Clinc. Pharmacol. 40: 513-519.

5. Gupta S.K., Manfro R.C., Tomlanovich S.J., Gambertoglio J.G., Garovoy M.R. and Benet L.Z., (1990): J. Clin. Pharmacol. 30: 643-653.
6. Rosano T.G., (1985): Clin. Chem. 31: 410-412.
7. Legg B. and Rowland M. (1987): J. Pharm. Pharmacol. 39: 599-603.
8. Gurecki J., Warty V. and Sanghvi A. (1985): Transplant. Proc. 17: 1997-2002.
9. de Groen P.C. (1988): Mayo Clin. Proc. 63: 1012-1021.
10. Vadiei K., Lopez-Berestein G., Perez-Soler R. and Luke D.R. (1989): Intern. J. Pharmaceutics 57: 133-138.
11. Venkataramanan R., Starzl T.E., Yang S., Burckart G.J., Ptachcinski R.J., Shaw B.W., Iwatsuki S., Van Thiel D.H., Sanghvi A. and Seltmann H. (1985): Transplant. Proc. 17: 286-289.
12. Venkataramanan R., Burckart G.J., and Ptachcinski R.J. (1985): Seminars in Liver Disease 5: 357-368.
13. Maurer G. (1985): Transplant. Proc. 17 (Suppl.1): 19-26
14. Kunzendorf U., Brockmöller J., Jochimsen F., Roots I. and Offermann G. (1989): Lancet I: 734-735.
15. Grevel J., Napoli K.L., Welsh M.S., Atkinson N.E. and Kahan B.D., (1991) Pharm. Res. 8: 278-281.
16. Kunzendorf U., Brockmöller J., Jochimsen F., Roots I. and Offermann G. (1989): Transplantation 48: 531-532.
17. Grevel J., Welsh M.S. and Kahan B.D. (1989): Ther. Drug Monit. 11: 246-248.
18. Wilkinson G.R. and Shand D.G. (1975): Clin. Pharmacol. Ther. 18: 377-390.
19. Yee G.C., Kennedy M.S., Storb R. and Thomas E.D. (1984): Blood 64: 1277-1279.
20. Kahan B.D., Kramer W.G., Wideman C., Flechner S.M., Lorber M.I. and Van Buren C.T. (1986): Transplantation 41: 459-464.
21. Yee G.C., Lennon T.P., Gmur D.J., Kennedy M.S. and Deeg H.J. (1986): Clin. Pharmacol. Ther. 40: 438-443.
22. Yee G.C. and McGuire T.R. (1990): Clin. Pharmacokin. 19: 319-332.
23. Wagner K. and Neumayer H.H. (1985): Lancet II: 1355-1356.
24. Davidson I., Root P., Fry W.R., Sando Z., Wilms C., Coorpender L., Alway C. and Reisch J. (1989): Transplantation 48: 575-580.
25. Grevel J. and Kahan B.D. (1991): Ther. Drug Monit. 13: 89-95.

CYCLOSPORIN TOXICITY AND LIVER TRANSPLANTATION IN HIGH RISK PATIENTS

D. Galmarini, L.R. Fassati, G. Rossi, B. Gridelli, L. Caccamo, M. Colledan, M. Doglia, G. Ferla, A. Lucianetti, U. Maggi, G. Paone, P. Reggiani.

Introduction

In Italy, Cyclosporin (CYS) is the drug that is electively used, together with steroids, to prevent rejection after liver transplantation (OLTX). The early (i.e. hypertension, kidney failure) and late (i.e. gingival hypertrophy, hirsutism, lymphoma) side effects caused by CYS use are well recognized entities (1). The damage to the graft, during the early postoperative period, is difficult to demonstrate and analyze. The aim of the present study is to evaluate the incidence of early and late side effects in high risk patients that did not receive any other rejection prophylaxis regime (e.g. OKT3, ATG) but steroids and azathioprine.

Materials and Methods

As of June 1991, 136 OLTX were performed at our institution on 120 patients, 98 adults and 22 children, with end stage hepatic failure. Among these 78 patients (65%) were considered at high risk, in order to the presence of one of the following preoperative risk factors: renal failure, acute digestive bleeding at time of surgery, ascites and hydrothorax, serum bilirubin level over 40 mg%, coma, infection, cerebral cortical atrophy, pulmonary hypertension; previous upper abdomen surgery and portal thrombosis were not included as risk factors. The indications for the hepatic transplantation in high risk patients were: hepatic cirrhosis (47), biliary cirrhosis (13), fulminant hepatitis (8), biliary atresia (5), Wilson's disease (4), Byler's disease (1). High risk patients are compared to the remaining 42 patients defined as at low risk; their indications to liver replacement were: hepatic cirrhosis (20), biliary cirrhosis (7), fulminant hepatitis (2), liver cancer (7), Wilson's disease (2), Byler's disease (4). In all patients immunosuppression was maintained with double drug association (cyclosporine and low dose of steroids), and azathioprine was added when necessary. CYS first dose was intraoperatively given as 6 mg/Kg i.v., and the targeted blood level in the following days was near 800 ng/ml (RIA). CYS oral administration was introduced around the 15th postoperative day with 10 mg/Kg/day dosage.

Results

Out of 120 transplanted patients 76 (63,3%) are alive with a mean follow up of 27 months. Common early side effects were: pulmonary infective complications, that appeared in 36% cases in high risk patients and in 20% in low risk; severe hypertension, that was present both in high risk (78%) and in low risk patients (70%), but in the first group it was particularly difficult to control and was cause of death for brain hemorrhage in two patients; maniac lethargic psychosis, almost lasting one week, that was present in 15% in high risk patients and 9% in low risk group; seizures, always successfully treated with barbiturates, that appeared in 7% of high risk patients versus 2% of the low risk patients. Other severe early side effects were present in the high risk group alone: kidney failure with oligo-anuria (20%), that required hemodialisis or ultrafiltration in 12 patients (15%); hemolysis, regressing with CYS withdrawal, in one patient; systemic Epstein-Barr virus infection, 45 days following liver

D. Galmarini et al. (eds.), Drugs and the Liver: High Risk Patients and Transplantation, 31–32.

transplantation, causing death in a patient that also received OKT3 therapy for acute rejection.

Bacterial, viral and fungal infections were equally present in high risk patients (29%) and low risk patients (33%), but they often were cause of death in the first group. Severe bacterial infections occurred in 10 high risk patients, being lethal in seven cases, versus 6 low risk patients, always recovered. Viral disease, by citomegalovirus (5 cases) and Epstein-Barr virus (1 case) had been shown in 6 patients from high risk group (4 death) versus 3 citomegalovirus recovered ones in the low risk group. Systemic fungal infections, all by Aspergillus fumigatus, were all fatal for 7 high risk patients, while were successfully recovered in 5 low risk patients.

As late side effects of CYS gingival hypertrophy and hirsutism were more or less present in all patients. Herpes Zoster virus infection occurred in 3 patients from the high risk group and in 1 case in the low risk group. Two cases of Kaposi's disease had been shown: two years after surgery for a high risk patient, who underwent acute rejection after CYS withdrawal and subsequently died for necrotizing pancreatitis, and 5 months after transplantation in a low risk patient, who developed an acute rejection episode after CYS interruption that caused the re-administration of CYS. Among low risk patients a colonic cancer and a lung tuberculosis occurred in the late follow up, 16 and 6 months respectively.

Discussion

Early side effects were almost widely present in high risk patients, while were less constant in low risk patients. Therefore major early complications appeared to be related to the severity of the preoperative clinical status, with particular regard to the kidney and lungs functions. Hemodialisis or ultrafiltration were be necessary only in the high risk patients with a 15% rate of incidence. In 11 high risk patients (14%) a prolonged ventilatory assistance was required because of various pulmonary infections. This was directly related to the death risk, as expressed by the fact that within the first two postoperative months high risk patients showed an infection related mortality (23%) higher than that of the low risk patients (2%).

In all our transplanted patients a similar incidence of early neurological minor complications and late side effects were evident. Late complications did not appear to be related to the pre-transplant conditions.

References

1) Kahan BD, Flechner SM, Lorber MI, Jensen C, Golden D, Van Buren CT. Complications of Cyclosporin therapy. World J Surg 1986; 10: 348-360.

DRUG TREATMENT IN LIVER TRANSPLANTED PATIENTS: ANTIHYPERTENSIVE THERAPY

Gastone Leonetti and Alberto Zanchetti

During the last decades the number of organs transplantation is significantly increased due to the widespread availability of effective immunosuppressing agents. However these procedures are responsible, in a certain meaning, of new clinical situation and among these the treatment of arterial hypertension in transplanted patients.

When we speak about treatment of arterial hypertension in liver transplanted patients we must distinguish (Table I) between arterial hypertension pre-existing to liver transplant, arterial hypertension following liver transplant and finally pre-existing arterial hypertension exacerbated by organ transplant.

Table I
ARTERIAL HYPERTENSION AND ORGAN TRANSPLANTATION

1) PRE-EXISTING HYPERTENSION

2) FOLLOWING TRANSPLANTATION

3) PRE-EXISTING AND WORSENED BY TRANSPLANTATION

Hypertension pre-existing to organ transplant In patients with arterial hypertension pre-existing to liver transplantation the antihypertensive treatment could be theoretically left unchanged, but, more theoretically than pragmatically (Table II). Indeed the liver is foundamental for the pharmakinetic profile of many antihypertensive drugs, because it may interfere on the bioavailability of drugs through the "hepatic first pass effect", on the transformation of inactive pro-drugs to active drugs and finally on the elimination phase of either the parent drugs or of their metabolites.

Many drugs, as for example beta-blockers and calcium-antagonists, have a very high degree of "hepatic first pass effect" which significantly decreases the amount of active drug which

D. Galmarini et al. (eds.), Drugs and the Liver: High Risk Patients and Transplantation, 33–41.

reaches the circulating blood.

Table II
ARTERIAL HYPERTENSION AND LIVER TRANSPLANTATION

1) HEPATIC FIRST-PASS EFFECT

2) PRO-DRUG ACTIVATION

3) BILIARY EXCRETION

4) HEPATIC TOXICITY

Therefore, if the liver function and the "first pass effect" is decreased, the dosage of antihypertensive agents should be lowered in order to avoid too high blood levels.

Some antihypertensive agents of the converting enzyme inhibitors family are orally administered as pro-drugs and are transformed to active drug at the hepatic level. In order to avoid the hepatic interference, the pro-drugs should be substituted by other antlhypertensive drugs of the same family which are administered as active drugs (and therefore do not need hepatic transformation) and are equally potent in blood pressure reduction.

The third aspect is the elimination of antihypertensive agents. Although the great majority of antihypertensive drugs have a renal clearance there are a few of them which have a biliary elimination. These agents again should be replaced in patients with liver transplantation by other antihypertensive agents with renal elimination or eventually should be administered at lower doses in order to avoid plasma accumulation.

Finally there are a few agents, as methyldopa, which may have a direct liver toxicity and these agents should be completely avoided.

From the pragmatic point of view all these pharmacokinetic aspects can be minimized either by replacing the agents with other antihypertensive agents with low first pass effect or active drugs, or by starting the antihypertensive therapy with lower doses and increasing thereafter the dosage according to the blood pressure reduction obtained and to the liver function tests.

Arterial hypertension following transplantation or exacerbated by transplantation A more interesting and new clinical situation is the development of arterial hypertension after organ transplantation or the worsening of a pre-existing hypertension and this problem has become more evident since the advent of cyclosporine in the armamentarium of immunosuppressive agents and therefore the remaining part will be concentrated on tne cyclosporine-associated hypertension as Porter has defined this medical situation in a recent work in the Archives of Internal Medicine (1).

At present time there are only a few data on cyclosporine-associated hypertension in liver transplanted patients (2) and the majority of data, which may help us to understand the mechanisms and treatment of the blood pressure elevation in cyclosporine treated patients, comes from kidney and bone-marrow transplantations and to a minor degree from patients who received cyclosporine for autoimmune disease as multiple sclerosis, posterior uveitis, primary biliary cirrhosis, rheumatoid arthritis, insulin-dependent diabetes (3).

1) Incidence of cyclosporine-associated hypertension. The most frequent transplants are those of the kidney, but this kind of transplantation may confound the interpretation of the incidence of cyclosporine-associated hypertension, because hypertension frequently coexists in patients with end-stage renal disease (4). However, in spite of this limitation, the incidence of cyclosporine-associated hypertension seems higher than that with other immunosuppressive drugs. Indeed, according to 3 prospective trials (5-7) the incidence of cyclosporine-associated hypertension in transplanted patients was higher (70.4%) than in patients who received the azathioprene-prednisone association (48.8%). However, in these patients high initial doses of cyclosporine were administered and the subsequent reduction of initial cyclosporine doses significantly lowered the development of hypertension. Furthermore, Kahan (8) has found that the incidence of hypertension decreases from very high percentages after 1 month (72%) to progressively lower incidences thereafter, being only 19% 2-3 years after transplantation.

According to Shorn (9), the incidence of hypertension in kidney transplant significantly increased from 71 to 85% in cyclosporine-prednisone treated patients, while in the azathioprene-prednisone group the incidence of hypertension decreased from 68 to 53%, confirming the association between cyclosporine and hypertension, independently from the transplanted organ.

This aspect (cyclosporine-associated hypertension) is more evident in patients undergoing bone-marrow transplant, that is in patients with normal liver and kidney function. Indeed Loughram (10) in a randomized prospective study has reported a 57% incidence of hypertension in cyclosporine treated patients versus only 4% in methotrexate-treated patients.

2) Clinical characteristics of cyclosporine-associated hypertension. The occurrence of cyclosporine-associated hypertension is unrelated to age, sex or race, while pre-existing hypertension may be accelerated by cyclosporine treatment (Table III). Hypertension is generally of mild and moderate degree and is on the whole asymptomatic; only rarely it may rapidly develop to severe hypertension and encephalopathy. In patients with liver transplant (11), toxic effects and hypertension during cyclosporine treatment were associated with low total cholesterol levels (below 120 mg/dl), while in patients with bone-marrow transplantation (12) lower serum magnesium levels were found. Finally a suppression of plasma renin activity and expansion of extracellular volume characterize the humoral pattern of cyclosporine-associated hypertension, which can be described as a volume-dependent rather than a renin-angiotensin-dependent form of hypertension (13-15).

Table III
CYCLOSPORINE-ASSOCIATED HYPERTENSION: CLINICAL CHARACTERISTICS

1) UNRELATED TO AGE, SEX AND RACE
2) GENERALLY OF MILD AND MODERATE DEGREE
3) SUPPRESSED PLASMA RENIN ACTIVITY
4) LOW SERUM MAGNESIUM LEVELS
5) LOW TOTAL CHOLESTEROL LEVELS IN LIVER TRANSPLANTATION

3) *Potential mechanisms of cyclosporine-associated hypertension.* All what we have reported until now on the cyclosporine-associated hypertension is indicative of a iatrogenic pathogenesis of blood pressure elevation. It should be therefore interesting and useful to understand the mechanisms underlying this association.

Among the potential mechanisms which may contribute to the development of hypertension or worsening of a pre-existing hypertension in cyclosporine-treated patients, we shall consider the nephrotoxic effects "di per se" (3) and the renal vasoconstriction, which has been documented in animals (16,17) and humans (18).

The renal vessels constriction can be mediated (Table IV) by a) stimulation of renal sympathetic nervous system, b) imbalance in the production of renal vasoconstrictor (eicosanoids) and vasodilator substances (prostaglandin synthesis), c) alteration of the renin-angiotensin-aldosterone system and d) finally a direct vascular effect due to interference with normally occurring mediator such as endothelial-derived relaxing factor (under this aspect are very interesting the recent reports which suggest that endothelial cells of microvessels are directly and in a very early phase involved in the graft rejection).

Table IV
CYCLOSPORINE-ASSOCIATED HYPERTENSION POTENTIAL MECHANISMS

1) NEPHROTOXIC EFFECTS

2) RENAL VASOCONSTRICTION
   a- stimulation of renal S.N.S.
   b- imbalance production of renal vasocostricting and vasodilating substances
   c- alteration of renin-angiotensin-aldosterone system
   d- direct vascular effect (interference with EDRF and/or endothelin)

a) Nephrotoxicity and hypertension in cyclosporine-treated patients. There are some controversial results among the studies concerning the role of nephrotoxic effect as a mechanism responsible of cyclosporine-associated hypertension. Indeed both nephrotoxic effects and hypertension may be present in cyclosporine-treated patients at therapeutic concentrations of the drug. All these data can explain that while hypertension is to be expected in patients with cyclosporine-associated renal dysfunction, the corollary, that hypertension is always associated with cyclosporine-caused renal dysfunction, is not true. The nephrotoxic pattern is characterized by marked reduction of glomerular filtration rate and renal plasma flow and tubulo-interstial damage, responsible of high sodium reabsorption.

However, according to some studies, if one compares the frequency of chronic cyclosporine nephrotoxic effects and the incidence of elevated blood pressure, the incidence of hypertension substantially exceeds that of nephrotoxic effects.

On the other side Dieterle in a recent review (3) on the incidence of nephrotoxic effects and hypertension in patients with autoimmune diseases treated with cyclosporine for up to 3 years found a parallel decrease in renal function (-17%) and a rise in blood pressure during the first 6 months of therapy and both the events levelled off after 4 months of cyclosporine therapy. He was able to identify some factors which seemed to influence the severity of long-term nephrotoxic effects, that is: 1) higher initial doses of cyclosporine and blood concentrations correlated with more profound decrease in creatinine clearance; 2) patients older than 60 years had a more profound decrease in creatinine clearance and 3) patients with rheumatoid arthritis and posterior uveitis appeared to be at greater risk of severe toxic effects. Monotherapy with cyclosporine, that is without corticosteroids in autoimmune disorders, is associated with hypertension and this is a further demonstration of the direct relationship between cyclosporine and hypertension.

In humans Loughram, as already mentioned, (10) found that 57% of patients treated with cyclosporine and only 4% of patients treated with methotrexate developed diastolic blood pressure greater than 90 mmHg. Clapman (19) reported similar findings of blood pressure elevations without clinically detectable changes in renal function.

b) Direct vasoconstriction of cyclosporine. These results suggest therefore that other mechanisms of cyclosporine-associated hypertension have to be identified and the possibility of direct renal vasoconstric- tion of cyclosporine has received special attention as potential explanation of this kind of hypertension.

Although the evidence for a role of the sympathetic nervous system in the cyclosporine-induced renal vasoconstriction has been supported by Murray (16) in animal experiments when he found that it was possible to reduce nephrotoxic effect with alpha-blockade or renal denervation, normal urinary excretion of catecholamines has been reported in cardiac transplant recipients who have been treated with cyclosporine. Furthermore Steigerwalt (21) found a reduction in plasma catecholamines and an increase in alpha-adrenergic receptors density in patients with cyclosporine-associated hypertension, which are exactly opposite results of what would be predicted if sympathetic nervous system would have played a significant contribution to cyclosporine-associated hypertension.

The possibility of an imbalance of arachidonic acid pathway has been suggested by animal experiments. Coffman (22) indeed found a significant increase in tromboxane production and a partial regression of cyclosporine induced renal vasoconstriction by blocking the tromboxane receptors or by inhibiting tromboxane production. Furthermore a synthetic prostaglandin E analogue (misoprostol) is able to overcome cyclosporine-induced renal vasoconstriction in rats (23).

Although acute animal experiments had shown a direct relationship between cyclosporine administration and stimulation of plasma renin activity (16,24), subsequent studies in humans have consistently shown a suppressed renin-angiotensin system, extracellular volume expansion and a sodium avid state in transplant recipients treated with cyclosporine (13,15,25). Furthermore in animal studies converting enzyme inhibitors did not reverse the cyclosporine-induced renal vasoconstriction.

In spite of these results we must be very careful in extrapolating the observed renal vasoconstriction to increased blood pressure, that is to systemic hemodynamic pattern, although it has been shown in spontaneous hypertensive rats (SHR) that cyclosporine causes increased vascular sensitivity to humoral and neurogenic stimuli. Finally, an interference of cyclosporine on the endothelial-derived relaxing factor or on the recently described endothelin, a potent endothelial derived vasoconstrictor substance, could be potential mechanisms of the cyclosporine-associated hypertension.

4) Therapeutic implications. The lack of conclusive results regarding the mechanism responsible of cyclosporine-associated hypertension does not allow the development of a rationale approach to therapy.

a) If cyclosporin-associated hypertension is sodium-dependent, as extracellular volume expansion would suggest, then diuretics and sodium restriction would be appropriate; however the potential substantial risk of volume depletion, enhancing nephrotoxic effects, is worrisome, particularly in renal transplant recipients.

b) It has been shown that cyclosporine binds to an intracellular calcium binding protein (cyclophilin) (26) and this could support a therapeutic approach to cyclosporine-associated hypertension with calcium-antagonists.

Bellet (20) has reported in human studies a significantly greater blood pressure reduction in cyclosporine-associated hypertension with the use of nifedipine than with captopril. More recently Curtis (reported in 1) has confirmed in a cross-over study that nifedipine 10 mg tid induced a greater reduction in both elevated blood pressure and renal vascular resistances than did captopril (this could be, also an indirect proof of a parallel renal and systemic cyclosporine-mediated vasoconstriction). In these patients captopril caused a small (5%), but significant decline in glomerular filtration rate. Finally, calcium-antagonists have a drug interaction with cyclosporine which raises blood levels of cyclosporine, possibly resulting in comparable immuno-suppression at lower cyclosporine dosages (27).

On the contrary the concurrent administration of steroids and non-steroidal anti-inflammatory drugs may complicate treatment because of their effects on blood volume and potential interference with the blood pressure lowering action of antihypertensive drugs.

Conclusion When one affords the problem of antihypertensive treatment in patients with liver or other organs transplantation he must differentiate between pre-existing and post-transplantation hypertension. In the first case one can use the classic first step antihypertensive agents, taking into account the specific details concerning the pharmacokinetic profile of the drug and potential liver toxicity. In post-transplant hypertension, frequently associated to cyclosporine treatment, calcium-antagonists appear to-day the most suitable agents while diuretics and converting enzyme inhibitors are the alternative or the associated antihypertensive drugs.

References

1. Porter GA, Bennet WB, Sheps SG. Cyclosporine-associated hypertension. Arch Intern Med 1990;150:280-3.
2. Krom RA. Liver transplantation at the Mayo Clinic. Mayo Clin Proc 1986;61:278-82.
3. Dieterle A, Abeywickrama K, Von-GraffenRied B. Nephrotoxicity and hypertension in patients with autoimmune disease treated with cyclosporine. Transplant Proc 1988;20 (suppl 4):349-55.
4. Weidle PJ, Vlasses PH. Systemic hypertension associated with cyclosporine: a review. Drug Intell Clin Pharm 1988;22:443-50.
5. McMaster P, Haynes IG, Michael J. Cyclosporine in cadaveric transplantation: a prospective randomized trial. Transplant Proc 1983;15 (suppl 1):2523-7.
6. The Canadian Multicenter Transplant Study Group. A randomized trial of cyclosporine in cadaveric renal transplantation. N Engl J Med 1983;309:809-15.
7. Sutherland DER, Fryd DS, Straud MH et al. Results of the Minnesota randomized prospective trial of cyclosporine versus azathioprine antilymphocyte globulin for immunosuppression in renal allograft recipients. Am J Kidney Dis 1985;5:318-27.
8. Kahan BD, Flechner SM, Lorber MI, Golden D, Conley S, VanBuren CT. Complication of cyclosporine-prednisone immunosuppression in 402 renal-allograft recipients exclusively followed at a single center for from 1 to 5 years. Transplantation 1987;43:197-204.
9. Schorn T, Frei U, Brackmann H, et al. Cyclosporine associated post-transplant hypertension: incidence and effect on renal transplant function. Transplant Proc 1988;20 (suppl 3):610-14.
10. Loughran TP, Deeg HJ, Dahlbuy S, Kennedy MS, Starb R, Thomas ED. Incidence of hypertension after marrow transplant among 112 patients randomized to either cyclosporine or nethotrexate as graft-versus host disease prophylaxis. Br J Haematol 1985;59:547-53.
11. DeGroen PC. Central nervous system toxicity after liver transplant: the role of cyclosporine and cholesterol. N Engl J Med 1987;317:861-6.
12. June CH, Thompson CB, Kennedy MS, Loughran TPJr, Deeg HJ. Correlation of hypomagnesemia with the onset of cyclosporine-associated hypertension in marrow transplant patients. Transplantation 1986;41: 47-51.
13. Bantee JP, Nath KA, Sutherland DE, Najaran JS, Ferris TF. Effects of cyclosporine on the renin-angiotensin system and potassium excretion in renal transplant patients. Arch Intern

Med 1985;145:505-8.
14. Bantee JP, Bovareau RJ, Ferris TP. Suppression of plasma renin activity by cyclosporine. Am J Med 1987;83:59-64.
15. Curtis JJ, Luke RG, Jones D, Diethelm AG. Hypertension in cyclosporine-treated renal transplant recipients is sodium dependent. Am J Med 1988;85:134-8.
16. Murray BM, Paller MS, Ferris TE. Effects of cyclosporine administration on renal hemodynamics in the conscious rat. Kidney Internat 1985;28:767-74.
17. English J, Evan A, Houghton DC, Bennett WM. Cyclosporine-induced renal dysfunction in the rat: evidence for arteriolar vasoconstriction with preservation of tubular function. Transplantation 1987;44: 135-41.
18. Curtis JJ, Luke RG, Dubousky E, Diethelm AG, Whelchel JD, Jones P. Cyclosporine in therapeutic doses increases renal allograft vascular resistance. Lancet 1986;ii:477-9.
19. Chapman JR, Macceu R, Arias M, Raine AE, Dunnill MS, Morris PJ. Hypertension after renal transplantation: a comparison of cyclosporine and conventional immunosuppression. Transplantation 1987;43:860-4.
20. Bellett M, Cabrol C, Sassano P, Leger P, Corval P, Menard J. Systemic hypertension after cardiac transplantation: effects of cyclosporine on renin-angiotensin-aldosterone system. Am J Cardiol 1985;56:927-31.
21. Steigerwalt S, McCurdy R, Smith S, Lockette W. Sympathetic nervous system in cyclosporine hypertension. Transplant Proc 1988;20 (suppl 3):341-5.
22. Coffman IM, Carr AR, Yarger WF, Klotman PE. Evidence that renal prostaglandins and tromboxane production is stimulated in chronic cyclosporine nephrotoxicity. Transplantation 1987;43:382-5.
23. Paller MS. Effects of prostaglandin E_1 analog misoprostol reverse acute cyclosporine toxicity. Transplant Proc 1988;20:634-7.
24. Barroe E, Boim MA, Ajzarn H, Ramos OL, Schor N. Glomerular hemodynamics and hormonal participation in cyclosporine nephrotoxicity. Kidney Internat 1987;32:19-25.
25. Stanek B, Kovarik J, Rasoulz-Rockenschuab S, Silberbauer K. Renin-angiotensin system and vasopressin in cyclosporine-treated renal allograft recipients. Clin Nephrol 1987;28:186-9.
26. Hait WN, Harding MW, Handschumacher RE, Colombani PM, Hess AD. Technical comments: calmodulin, cyclophilin and cyclosporine A. Science 1986;233:987-9.
27. Pochert JM, Pirson Y. Cyclosporine-diltiazem interaction. Lancet 1986;i: 979 (abstract)

BACTEREMIA AFTER LIVER TRANSPLANTATION; FEW ISSUES IN SELECTION OF ANTIBIOTICS FOR TREATMENT AND PROPHYLAXIS

S. Kusne, M. Alessiani, M. Martin, J. Fung, T.E. Starzl

Infections after liver transplantation are still associated with significant morbidity and mortality. Bacterial infections account for up to 50% of such events according to various series. The majority of these infections are nosocomial and many of them are associated with technical surgical problems. Bacteremia represents "invasive" infection and knowing the common agents involved helps in selection of antibiotics for treatment and prophylaxis. Successful use of antibiotics requires familiarity with their characteristics, potential side effects and interactions with other medications.

COMMON BACTEREMIAS

In a previous study from our institution, we had a frequency of bacteremia of 26%, occurring after liver transplantation in 101 consecutive patients (1). All 33 bacterial isolates in that study are shown in table 1. Fifty one percent of episodes of bacteremia with a single isolate were due to gram negative enteric organisms, and only 27% to gram positive isolates. This is in contrast to what has been published by other centers that routinely use selective bowel decontamination in liver transplantation. In one study 81% of bacteremias were caused by gram positive organisms and only 6% by gram negatives (2). Anaerobes account for a very small portion of bacterial infections after liver transplantation in any center. This information is important for selection of empiric antibiotics in the septic patient. Empiric antibiotic coverage depends on the suspected source for bacteremia. For example, if cholangitis is suspected coverage should

D. Galmarini et al. (eds.), Drugs and the Liver: High Risk Patients and Transplantation, 43–47.

include gram negative enteric organisms and enterococci; if intravascular lines or wound infection is suspected staphylococcus coverage should be considered.

The most common source of bacteremia after liver transplantation is the abdomen and this is often related to surgical/or mechanical problems (surgical wounds, hepatic artery thrombosis and other vascular complications, biliary obstruction and leaks etc). Most bacteremias occur during the first two months after transplantation (primary or retransplantation), and in our original study 61% of thirty three bacteremias followed this rule.

SELECTION OF ANTIBIOTICS FOR PROPHYLAXIS

Perioperative antibiotic coverage for liver transplantation should include gram negative organisms and enterococci. In our institution we use cefotaxime or ceftizox in combination with ampicillin for the duration of 72 hours. Trimethoprim/sulfamethoxazole given for prevention of pneumocystis carinii pneumonia may also have an effect on prevention of bacterial infections. The routine use of selective bowel decontamination is practiced by some centers. The literature does not show clearly that there is an advantage to its use since:
a. although infections caused by gram negative bacteria are low those caused by gram positive bacteria are higher, b. there is no difference in overall mortality and Intensive Care Unit stay, c. the emergence of resistant organisms is a possibility (3).

OTHER FACTORS IMPORTANT IN SELECTION OF ANTIBIOTICS

Cholangitis

It accounts for 6-10% of bacterial infections after transplantation and is associated with bacteremia in about 40%. Diagnosis is usually difficult due to the fact that biliary draining tubes (like T-tube) are often colonized with bacteria, inflammatory white cells are not easily recognized in bile and the latter is not always available for culture. Therefore empiric antibiotics should be started whenever there is clinical suspicion of bacterial cholangitis. The clinician should be familiar with the fact that some antibiotics do not penetrate well in bile (4). For example Imipenem/ Cilastatin has a very broad antibacterial coverage but penetrates bile very poorly, if at all. Cholangitis is usually associated with biliary obstruction which imply no penetration of antibiotics to bile, until obstruction is relieved. Some authors feel that serum concentration of antibiotics is as important as biliary penetration. Although the most common antibiotics used in cholangitis are ampicillin or cephalosporins in combination with aminoglycoside, the ureido-penicillins (like mezlocillin, azlocillin and piperacillin) with or without aminoglycosides may have very important role because of their good biliary penetration.

Hepatotoxicity

Antibacterial agents prescribed after liver transplantation may be toxic to the new allograft. Medications prescribed for treatment and prevention of tuberculosis (like isoniazid, pyrazinamide and rifampin) may cause hepatitis. Hypersensitivity reactions with liver enzymes elevation can be seen with erythromycin and sulfonamides. SGOT elevation at times self limited can be seen with use of commonly prescribed antibiotics (like carbenicillin, cloxacillin, moxalactam etc.).

Bleeding

Some beta-lactam antibiotics may affect coagulation and cause bleeding. One mechanism which causes hypoprothrombinemia is probably through interference with vitamin k metabolism (5). This is described with cephalosporins that have Methyl-thio-tetrazole side chain (like cefamandole, moxalactam and cefoperazone). A second mechanism results in platelets dysfunction and is described with antibiotics like ticarcillin, piperacillin and mezlocillin. This is important to remember since these patients may have coagulation abnormalities secondary to liver disease.

Nephrotoxicity

The aminoglycosides are the main antibiotics to cause nephrotoxicity after liver transplantation. They usually damage the proximal tubules causing non-oliguric renal failure. This is more pronounced when an aminoglycoside is prescribed together with vancomycin. Some authors feel that there is increased risk of renal dysfunction due to interaction of liver disease and the aminoglycosides (6). Obviously when the clinician can choose non nephrotoxic antibiotic it is preferable, but in some infections (like enterococcus sepsis) there is no "other choice".

Interaction with other drugs

Before prescribing any antibiotics or antimicrobials in patients after transplantation one has finally to consider possible interactions with other medications. The interactions of Cyclosporin (Cya) with antimicrobials were summarized by others (7). Through inhibition or induction of hepatic P-450 enzyme system some agents can increase and others can lower Cya levels. Erythromycin and ketoconazole can increase Cya level causing nephrotoxicity while rifampin can significantly lower Cya level leading to rejection of the allograft.

TABLE 1: All 33 bacteremia isolates that occurred in 101 consecutive liver transplant patients.

BACTERIA INVOLVED (No; %)	NUMBER EPISODES
Gram Negative Bacteremia (17; 51)	
Pseudomonas aeruginosa	7
Escherichia coli	4
Klebsiella pneumoniae	3
Citrobacter freundii	2
Enterobacter cloacae	1
Gram Neg./Pos. Bacteremia (4; 12)	
Gram Positive Bacteremia (9; 27)	
Enterococcus	4
Staphylococcus epidermidis	2
Staphylococcus aureus	1
Streptococcus bovis	1
Listeria monocytogenes	1
Anaerobic Bacteremia (3; 9)	
Bacteroides fragilis	2
Clostridia species	1

REFERENCES

1. Kusne S, Dummer JS, Singh N, Singh, N, Iwatsuki I, Makowka L, Esquivel C, Tzakis AG, Starzl TE, Ho M (1988): Medicine 67: 132.
2. Paya CV, Herman PE, Washington II JA, Smith TF, Anhalt JP, Wiesner RH, Krom R. (1989) Mayo Clin Proc 64: 555.
3. Martin M, Kusne S, Alessiani M, Simmons R, Starzl T. (1991) Transplant Proc 23: 1929.

4. Munro R, Sorrell TC, Drugs (1986) 31: 449
5. Sattler FR, Weitekamp MR, Ballard JO, Ann Intern Med (1986) 105: 924.
6. Moore RD, Smith CR, Lietman PS, Am J Med (1986) 80: 1093
7. Sands M, Brown RB, (1989) Rev Infect Dis 11: 691.

ANTIVIRAL DRUGS

F. Dianzani, G. Antonelli.

The peculiarity of viruses among the microorganisms is their extreme dependence on the metabolic and biosinthetics apparatuses of the host cell. Since a virus must grow within the host cell, it must be viewed together with its host in any consideration concerning therapy, host defense, pathogenesis, or epidemiology.

Viruses are difficult targets for chemotherapy because, as already stated, they replicate only within host cells, mainly utilizing many of the host cell's biosynthetic processes. The similarity of host-directed and virus-directed processes makes it difficult to find antiviral agents specific enough to exert a greater effect on viral replication in infected cells than on functions of uninfected host cells. In fact since the last decade it became evident that only a few steps of the life cycle of each particular virus could form the basis for useful design of chemotherapeutic agents. Additionally many of the antiviral compounds that have been developed <u>in vitro</u> are not effective <u>in vivo</u> or, more importantly and frequently, have a narrow ratio of efficacy to toxicity. It is becoming increasingly apparent, however, that each virus may have a few specific steps of replication that may be used as targets for highly selective, carefully aimed chemotherapeutic agents. Proper use of such drugs requires a profound knowledge of the suitable targets, based on correct diagnosis and precise understanding of the replicative mechanism of the offending virus. For instance in the case of AIDS, a widely explored area as far as chemotherapy is concerned, some steps of HIV replication have been identified as potential targets for antiviral drugs, (namely: attachment; transcription of viral RNA to

D. Galmarini et al. (eds.), Drugs and the Liver: High Risk Patients and Transplantation, 49–54.

proviral DNA; proteolytic cleavage of the viral precursor protein; assembly and release of mature virions). Conversely only one possible target has been so far identified for herpes simplex virus (viral DNA polymerase). For each of these steps specific compounds have been developed which can be clinically useful.

However, among the number of substances which have been shown to be active in vitro only a few compounds have been approved for therapeutic use.

Table 1 summarizes the molecular target and therapeutical indications of the main agents approved for clinical use.

TABLE 1. Main antiviral agents approved for therapy of viral diseases.

Compound (ref.)	Main target	Main indications (infection by)
-Amantadine(1)	penetration or uncoating*	influenza A virus
-Rimantadine(2)	as above	influenza A virus
-Acyclovir(3)	viral-DNA polymerase	HSV VZV
-ARA A(4)	as above	HSV
-Ganciclovir(5)	as above	cytomegalovirus
-Ribavirin(6)	viral-RNA polymerase guanylil-transferase	influenza A virus RSV Lassa virus
-AZT(7-9)	reverse transcriptase	HIV
-Iododeoxy uridine(10,11)	viral DNA synthesis	HSV
-Trifluoro thymidine(12)	as above	HSV

HSV=Herpes simplex virus; RSV=respiratory sincityal virus; HIV=human immunodeficiency virus; VZV=Varicella zoster virus; AZT=azidothymidine; ARA A= adenine arabinoside or vidarabine.

*In some cases an inhibitory effect on viral assembly has been demonstrated.

It should be mentioned that among the compounds shown in the table only acyclovir, and at a lesser extent AZT and ganciclovir meet the characteristics of the ideal antiviral agents. Particurarly, acyclovir which is a guanosine analog [specifically: 9-(2-hydroxy ethoxymethil guanine)], is the first antiviral agent which needs a viral enzyme (the viral thymidine kinase) to be effectively activated.

This enzyme, obviously present only in infected cells, phosphorylates acyclovir which in turn inhibits the viral DNA polymerase. It is worth noting that once phosphorylated acyclovir has a much higher affinity for viral DNA polymerase as compared to cellular DNA polymerase, thus further explaining the high ratio of efficacy to toxicity of this compound. Similarly, although at lesser extent, also AZT, which is a thymidine analog (specifically: 3'-Azido-3' -deoxythymidine), is selective since its affinity for viral reverse transcriptase is much higher than that for cellular DNA polymerase.

It should be pointed out, however, that even selective drugs such as AZT or acyclovir can cause, when administered in man for long periods of time, serious side effects (such as anemia and renal dysfunction,respectively) or can easily select pharmaco-resistant viral mutants. For instance AZT-resistant variant of HIV-1 was obtained in our laboratory by growing HTLV-IIIB strain of HIV-1 in C8166 cells, a CD4+ lymphoblastoid cell line very sensitive to HIV-1 infection (13), in the presence of inhibitory concentrations of AZT. The resistant strain was capable of replicating, as measured by infectious virus yield (table 2) and inducing cytophatic effect in the presence of AZT concentrations able to completely suppress the replication of parental HTLV-IIIB. Cloning of this resistant population revealed that a number of different variants of HIV-1 with various degrees of sensitivity to AZT may be generated during propagation of HTLV-IIIB in C8166 cells in the presence of the drug (data not shown).

Beside to classical chemotherapeutic agents there are several other "physiologic" agents which can be considered antiviral agents. These substances (such as interferons, cytokines and immunomodulators) may directly affect viral replication or may undirectly increase cellular or humoral immunity of the host against viral diseases. Some of them, i.e. interferons (IFNs), are being used as therapeutic agents in several infections and have found well established therapeutic applications. These proteins are naturally produced body products that are mainly involved in the regulation of the host-defense mechanism as well as in the homeostatic regulation of growth and differentiation. They represent the body's most rapid defence against virus infections. Natural recovery from viral infections is correlated with IFN production. In fact the inhibition of IFN production or action enhances the severity of infection; conversely, IFN administration has been shown to protect animals from several viral infections.

Table 2. AZT-resistance of HIV-R1 as measured by viral yield.

Virus	Viral yield (Log TCID50/ml) in the presence of AZT (uM):				
	5.0	0.5	0.05	0.005	0
HTLV-IIB	<1.5	<1.5	2.8	4.8	5.6
HIV-R1	3.3	4.2	6.1	5.8	6.2

HIV-R1 was obtained after propagation of HTLV-IIIB in C8166 cells in the presence of AZT. C8166 cells were infected with HTLV-IIIB or HIV-1 at the same m.o.i. in the presence or absence of different concentrations of AZT; viral progeny was measured 48 hrs later. Basically the same results were obtained in three additional experiments.

The IFNs are, on the basis of antigenicity and molecular structure divided into three main classes; alpha, beta and gamma (14). IFN beta is produced by fibroblasts in response to viral infections. IFN alpha or leucocyte IFN may be induced by foreign or infected cells or by viruses and it is continuously released into the bloodstream during infection, declining with time. IFN gamma is produced later by virus-sensitized T lymphocytes. The antiviral action of IFNs is induced by their interaction with specific receptors on the cell surface leading to translation of secondary antiviral proteins. IFNs may also enhance immune response by increasing expression of lymphocyte surface antigens and by increasing the cytotoxic activity of natural killer cells. Three main important properties of IFNs gave rise to their use in the therapy of viral and neoplastic diseases: high specific activity; low toxicity; pleiotropic effects (15). Since many studies have shown that IFNs may act as natural defense mechanism, it was tempting to speculate that IFNs could provide a means to control viral infections. Indeed, excellent to promising results have been reported on the use of IFN beta and IFN alpha in the therapy of viral diseases (table 3) or other diseases of unknown etiology whose connection with a viral infection has been postulated (multiple sclerosis, mycosis fungoides). It should be mentioned that, although originally unexpected, also IFN administration has been shown to be correlated with a number of side effects. Among them there is also the development of antibodies to IFN whose clinical significance is still to be clarified (16).

TABLE 3. Main therapeutical application of interferons against viral diseases.

Virus	Interferon type	Administration
Hepatitis B	alpha	s.c, or i.m.
C	alpha	s.c, or i.m.
D	alpha	s.c, or i.m.
Papovavirus	alpha, beta	topical,i.m.,i.l.
HSV	alpha, beta	topical, i.l.
Rhinovirus*	alpha	topical

* Only for prophylaxis. s.c.=subcutaneously; i.m.=intramuscolarly; i.l.= intralesional.

ACKNOWLEDGEMENTS.

This work was supported in part by a grant from Ministero della Sanità, Istituto Superiore di Sanita' (Progetto AIDS).

REFERENCES

1. Hay A.J., Wolstenholme A.J., Skehel J.J., Smith M.H. (1985): The molecular basis of the specific anti-influenza action of amantadine. Embo J., 4: 3021-3024.

2. Bukrinskaya A.G., Vorkunova N.K., Kornilayeva G.V., Vorkunova G.K.(1982): Influenza virus uncoating in infected cells and effect of rimantadine. J.Gen.Virol., 60: 49-59.

3. St.Clair M.H., Furman P.A., Lubbers C.M. Elion.B. (1980): Inhibition of cellular alpha and virally-induced deoxyribonucleic acid polymerase by the triphosphate of acyclovir. Antimicrob. Agents Chemother., 18: 741-74.

4. Shipman C., Smith S., Carlson R.H., Drach J.C. 1976): Antiviral activity of arabinosyladenine and arabinosylhypoxanthine in herpes simplex virus infected KB cells. Selective inhibition of viral DNA synthesis in synchronized suspension cultures. Antimicrob. Agents Chemother., 9: 120-127.

5. Field A.K., Davies M.E., Dewitt C.(1983): 9- 2-Hydroxy-1-(hydroxymethyl)ethoxy methyl guanine: A selective inhibitor of herpes group virus replication. Proc. Natl. Acad. Sci. USA, 80: 4139-

4143.
6. Cheng Y.C., Huang E.S., Lin J.C. (1983): Unique spectrum of activity of 9-(1,3-dihydroxy-2-propoxylmethyl)-guanine against herpes viruses in vitro and its mode of action against herpes simplex virus type 1. Proc.Natl. Acad. Sci. USA, 80: 2767-2770.
7. Mitsuya H., Weinhold K.J., Furman P.A. (1985): 3'-azido-3'-deoxythymidine (BWA509U): An antiviral agent that inhibits the infectivity and cytophatic effect of human T-lymphotropic virus type III/lymphoadenopathy-associated virus in vitro. Proc. Natl. Acad. Sci. USA, 82: 7096-7100.
8. Fischl M.A., Richman D.D., Grieco M.H.(1987): The efficacy of azidothymidine (AZT) in the treatment of patients with AIDS and AIDS-related complex-a double-blind placebo-controlled trial. N. Engl. J. Med., 317: 185-191.
9. Hirsch M.S.(1988): AIDS commentary-azidothymidine. J. Infect. Dis., 157: 427-431.
10. Kaufman H.E., Martola E.L., Dohlman C.I. (1962): Use of 5-iodo-2'-deoxyuridine (IDU) in treatment of herpes simplex keratitis. Arch. Ophthalmol., 68: 235-239.
11. Prusoff W.H. (1959).Synthesis and biological activation of iododeoxyuridine, an analog of thymidine. Biochim. Biophys. Acta, 32: 295-296.
12. Prusoff W.H., Mancini W.R., Lin T.S., Lee J.J., Siegel S.Z., Otto M.G.(1984): Physical and biological consequences of incorporation of antiviral agents into virus DNA. Antiv. Resear., 4:303-315.
13. Dianzani F., Antonelli G., Capobianchi M.R., De Marco F. (1988): Replication of human immunodeficiency virus: yield of infectious under single growth cycle conditions. Arch. Virol. 103: 127-131.
14. Dianzani F., Antonelli G., and Capobianchi M.R. (1990): The biological basis for clinical use of interferon. J. Hepatol. 11: S5-S10.
15. Baron S., Dianzani F., Stanton G.J., and Fleischmann R.W.Jr. editors (1987): The Interferon system: A current review to 1987. University of Texas press, Austin.
16. Antonelli G., Currenti M., Turriziani O., and Dianzani F. (1991): Neutralizing antibodies to Interferon: Relative frequency in patients treated with different Interferon preparations. J. Infect. Dis. 163: 882-885.

THE USE OF ANTIVIRAL DRUGS IN LIVER TRANSPLANT PATIENTS

T. Wreghitt

Virus infections are a significant cause of morbidity and mortality in liver transplant patients [1 - 3]. The incidence and severity of these infections in transplant patients is influenced by the severity of the basic immunosuppressive regime, the immunosuppressive agents used (particularly azathioprine, ATG, and OKT3), the rejection rates experienced and associated therapy, the prevalence of virus infections in the recipient and donor population, and, most significantly, the extent of donor/recipient virus mismatch (i.e. cytomegalovirus (CMV) antibody-positive donor and negative recipient). The age of the recipients and donors will also influence the incidence of virus infections.

Cytomegalovirus is the most important virus infecting liver transplant patients. Infection is associated with fever, malaise, leucopenia, gastrointestinal tract ulceration, confusion, arthritis, hepatitis, and the most feared complication, pneumonitis, which may be fatal.Severe symptoms are most commonly associated with donor/recipient CMV mismatch. Antiviral drugs are available for the treatment or prophylaxis of CMV infections [Table 1].

Herpes simplex virus (HSV) infections usually arise in the first few weeks after transplantation, when patients are most immunosuppressed. Infection may be associated with oro-facial lesions, genital lesions, mucositis, hepatitis and pneumonitis. Symptoms are usually mild and respond rapidly to acyclovir treatment, but severe symptoms may arise notably pneumonitis which may be fatal if not diagnosed promptly and treated with intravenous acyclovir. All HSV infections are reactivations of latent

D. Galmarini et al. (eds.), Drugs and the Liver: High Risk Patients and Transplantation, 55–60.

infection arising in patients who are HSV antibody positive before transplantation.

Epstein-Barr virus (EBV) infection is frequently found in transplant patients, but few infections are associated with severe symptoms. Patients may experience fever and hepatitis, particularly in donor-acquired primary infection. EBV may also be associated with a lymphoproliferative syndrome. The most serious result of EBV infection is lymphoma.

Varicella-zoster virus (VZV) is most commonly associated with reactivation of latent infection (zoster) in adult patients, 95% of whom will have had previous chickenpox. Primary infection (chickenpox) is most commonly found in paediatric patients, but cases do arise in adults. Both zoster and chickenpox may be associated with severe symptoms and are treated with acyclovir.

Adenovirus infections are usually associated with respiratory tract symptoms, but may also produce a morbilliform rash and hepatitis[1]. Adenovirus infections are found most frequently in paediatric patients. There is as yet no treatment available, but ganciclovir has *in vitro* activity and may be of some use clinically[4].

Hepatitis B (HBV) and hepatitis C (HCV) viruses may also be found in liver transplant patients but there is as yet no recommended antiviral drug regimes available for their treatment although ribavirin has shown promising results for treating hepatitis C virus infections.

ANTIVIRAL DRUGS

The antiviral drugs available for treating virus infections in transplant patients are shown in Table 1.

TABLE 1 Available antiviral drugs

Antiviral drug	Virus
Acyclovir	HSV, VZV, CMV
Ganciclovir	CMV
Foscarnet	CMV
Interferon	HBV, HCV
Ribavirin	HCV

Acyclovir

Acyclovir (Zovirax, Wellcome) is an acyclic analogue of 2[1] - deoxyguanosine. It acts as a DNA polymerase inhibitor and a chain terminator and is inactive unless phosphorylated by enzymes to acyclovir triphosphate. HSV and VZV thymidine kinases convert acyclovir to acyclovir monophosphate and by this means virus infected cells acquire a higher concentration of the drug than uninfected cells. Acyclovir monophosphate is converted to acyclovir diphosphate by cellular guanosine monophosphate kinase and other cellular enzymes convert this to acyclovir triphosphate.

Acyclovir is a safe and effective drug for treating HSV and VZV infections, with few side effects; most are reversible when the drug is withdrawn. Patients may experience temporary renal failure if too high a dose is given too quickly and nausea, vomiting, burns around infusion sites, and CNS symptoms may arise in a few patients. The drug is available in a number of formulations, but use in transplant patients usually involves oral and intravenous preparations. Seventy percent of acyclovir is excreted in the urine and the dose must be reduced in patients with renal impairment. Much higher doses have to be given orally because of poor absorption from the gut. Although acyclovir-resistant strains of virus may be found, these are uncommon and arise most frequently in patients on prolonged treatment.

Treatment and prophylaxis of HSV infections

Severe HSV infections should be treated with 10 mg/kg intravenous acyclovir three times a day for 7-10 days. Less serious infections may be treated with oral acyclovir (200-400 mg 4-5 times a day). The most serious form of HSV infection, pneumonitis, which may be fatal [5], must be treated with the intravenous dose above and in heart-lung transplant patients, we have found that patients should then receive prolonged oral acyclovir (200 mg 4 times a day) in order to minimize recurrent symptoms (5). Many transplant centres use acyclovir prophylactically in the first few months after transplantation in order to reduce the incidence and severity of HSV infections.

Treatment of VZV infections

Since chickenpox may be severe or fatal in transplant recipients[6] acyclovir (10 mg/kg three times a day) should be used for treatment. Zoster immune globulin should also be given. Patients with zoster should be given either oral acyclovir (800 mg five times a day) or intravenous acyclovir according to the severity of the symptoms.

Prophylaxis of CMV infections

Since acyclovir is of little benefit in treating CMV infections [7], its use is restricted to prophylaxis. Meyers *et al.* [8] demonstrated the beneficial effect of i.v. acyclovir in bone marrow transplant recipients with CMV disease. Balfour *et al* [9] reported that in a randomized, placebo-controlled trial, oral acyclovir (800 - 3200 mg a day for 12 weeks) reduced the rate of CMV infection and disease in kidney transplant recipients. The benefit of prophylactic acyclovir was greatest in CMV mismatched patients.

In a non-randomized clinical trial in CMV mismatched liver transplant recipients, Stratta *et al* [10] reported the beneficial effects of prophylactic i.v. immunoglobulin (0.5 g/kg at weekly intervals for six weeks) and i.v. acyclovir (5 mg/kg three times a day for 3 months). Twenty-one patients were historical controls and the next 21 received prophylaxis. The incidence of CMV disease was reduced from 71% to 24%.

Ganciclovir

Ganciclovir (Cymevene, Syntex) is an acyclic analogue of 2^1 - deoxyguanosine, and is similar in structure to acyclovir, but has an additional 3^1 carbon and hydroxyl group on the acyclic side chain which gives ganciclovir a 25 - 100fold enhanced efficacy against CMV compared with acyclovir. CMV enzymes convert ganciclovir to ganciclovir monophosphate, which is modified to ganciclovir triphosphate by host enzymes. Ganciclovir triphosphate inhibits CMV replication by selective inhibition of CMV DNA polymerase. Although ganciclovir is the drug of choice for treating CMV infections in transplant recipients, side effects, most notably neutropenia and thrombocytopenia may be found. Ganciclovir produces more side-effects than acyclovir. CNS symptoms, anaemia, fever, rash and raised liver enzymes may also be noted. In general, ganciclovir is well tolerated and few transplant patients experience sufficient side effects for treatment to be stopped. The recommended dose is 5 mg/kg twice a day i.v., but patients with renal impairment should receive lower doses. Although ganciclovir-resistant strains of CMV have been recovered, this is unusual unless patients are receiving prolonged treatment[11].

Treatment of CMV infections

CMV pneumonia is the most difficult CMV disease manifestation to treat and ganciclovir treatment in bone marrow transplant patients has been disappointing[12]. Crumpacker *et al.*[13] reported that 38% bone marrow transplant patients with CMV pneumonitis survived for at least 90 days on ganciclovir, however their patients also received CMV immunoglobulin which probably contributed in this uncontrolled trial to their better results. Paya *et al.*[14] noted marked clinical improvement in 5 of 6 liver transplant patients with CMV disease. In a study of ganciclovir treatment in liver, kidney and heart transplants with CMV disease, Dunn *et al.*[15] noted 30 day cure rates of 89%, although 21% patients required re-treatment subsequently. Shaefer *et al.*[16] recorded lasting cures in 70% of 84 liver transplant patients with CMV disease treated with one course of ganciclovir.

Prophylaxis of CMV infections

Schmidt *et al.*[17] demonstrated a beneficial effect of prophylactic ganciclovir in bone marrow transplant patients with CMV infection in a randomized controlled trial. Twenty-five percent of patients receiving ganciclovir died from CMV pneumonitis compared with 70% patients who were not given prophylaxis ($p = 0.01$). Initial results in solid organ transplant patients have been promising. It is probable that prophylaxis with either acyclovir or ganciclovir (maybe combined with CMV immunoglobulin which has been shown to be beneficial prophylactically) followed by treatment with ganciclovir in those patients who have laboratory evidence of active CMV infection will emerge as the management protocol.

REFERENCES

1. Wreghitt T.G., Hughes M. and Calne, R.Y. (1987): *Serodiag. Immunother.*,1: 219-39.
2. Dummer J.S., Hardy A., Poorsattar A. and Ho M. (1983): *Transplantation,* 36: 259-67.
3. Salt A., Sutehall G.A., Sargaisson M., Woodward C., Barnes N. D., Calne R. Y. and Wreghitt T.G. (1990): *J. Clin. Pathol.*, 43: 63-7.
4. Wreghitt, T.G., Gray J.J., Ward K.N., Salt A., Taylor D.L., Alp N.J. and Tyms A.S. (1989): *J. Inf.*, 19: 88-9.
5. Smyth R.L., Higenbottam T.W., Scott J.P., Wreghitt T.G., Stewart S., Clelland C.A., McGoldrick J.P. and Wallwork J. (1990): *Transplantation,* 49: 735-9.
6. Bradley J.R., Wreghitt T.G. and Evans D.B. (1987): *Nephrol. Dial. Transplant.,* 1: 242-5.
7. Balfour H.H. (1990): *Rev. Inf. Dis.,* 12 (suppl. 7): S849-60.
8. Meyers J.D., Reed E.C., Shepp D.H., Thornquist M., Dandliker P.S., Vicary C.A., Flournoy N., Kirk, L.E., Kersey J.H., Thomas E.D. and Balfour H.H. (1988): *N. Eng. J. Med.*, 318: 70-5.
9. Balfour H.H., Chace B.A., Stapleton J.T., Simmons R.L. and Fryd D.S.(1989): *N. Eng. J. Med.*, 320: 1381-7.
10. Stratta R.J., Shaefer M.S., Cushing K.A., Markin R.S., Wood R.P., Langnas A.N., Reed E.C., Woods G.L., Donovan J.P., Pillen T.J., Li S., Duckworth R.M. and Shaw B.W. (1991): *Transplantation,* 51: 90-7.
11. Erice A., Chou S., Biron K.K., Stanat S.C., Balfour H.H. and Jordan M.C. (1989): *N. Eng. J. Med.*, 320: 289-93.

12. Erice A., Jordan M.C., Chace B.A., Fletcher C., Chinnock B.J. and Balfour H.H. (1987): *J.A.M.A.*, 257: 3082-7
13. Crumpacker C., Marlowe S., Zhang J.L., Abrams S., Watkins P. and the Ganciclovir Bone Marrow Transplant Group. (1988): *Rev. Inf. Dis.*, 10 (Suppl. 3): S538-46.
14. Paya C.V., Hermans P.E., Wiesner R.H., Ludwig J., Smith T.F., Rakela J. and Krom R.A.F. (1989): *J. Inf. Dis.*, 160: 752-8.
15. Dunn D.L., Mayoral J.L., Gillingham K.J. Loeffler C.M., Brayman K.L., Kramer M.A., Erice A., Balfour H.H., Fletcher C.V., Bolman R.M., Matas A.J., Payne W.D., Sutherland D.E.R. and Najarian J.S. (1991): *Transplantation*, 51: 98-106.
16. Shaefer M.S., Stratta R.J., Markin R.S., Cushing K.A., Woods G.L., Reed E.C., Wood R.P., Langas A.N. and Shaw B.W. (1991): *Trans. Proc.*, 23: 1515-6.
17. Schmidt G.M., Horak D.A., Niland J.C., Duncan S.R., Forman S.J., Zaia J.A. and the City of Hope-Stanford-Syntex CMV Study Group. (1991): *N. Eng. J. Med.*, 324: 1005-11.

DRUGS, FETAL LIVER AND REPRODUCTION

P. V. Grella

As nearly all allograft patient require continuous immunosuppression to prevent organ rejection, it is important to understand the effects of immunosuppressive drugs may have on the mother and fetus.

All immunosuppressive drugs increase susceptibility to common infections, as well as opportunistic, bacterial, viral, and fungal. For example, more than 15% of renal transplant patients have bacteriuria, and approximately 5% may develop pyelonephritis, which may trigger sepsis or, in pregnancy, preterm labor. Consequently, it is very important to monitor the immunosuppressed pregnant patient for early signs and symptoms of infection.

Prolonged use of immunosuppressive agents may also increase the likelihood of neoplastic changes. Therefore, it is equally necessary to pay careful attention to cervical cytology, breast masses, and the hematologic profile in the pregnant transplant patient.

Pregnancy itself associated with important immunologic phenomena. The fetus, which can be considered as an allogenic graft, and grows in condition that contradict the usual laws of transplantation immunogenetics. The failure of rejection may be explained by a sequence of immunologic alterations: anatomic changes in the uterus render it a privileged site for the graft implantation and survival; absent or ineffective expression of transplantation antigens on the trophoblast; changes in maternal lymphocyte subset during pregnancy with diminished cellular immune response; separation of maternal and fetal circulation. The maternal immune system is depressed in certain cellular reactions and this is due to immunosuppressive factors in the mother's serum such as alpha-2-glycoproteins and various hormones rather than to intrinsic defects in the lymphocytes. Granulocyte chemotaxis was reported to be depressed when tested in the presence of pregnant women's serum.

The placenta facilitates the transport of IgG from the mother to the fetus, and at the same time it stops the transport of other immunoglobulin classes. Drugs given to the mother have variable capacity to cross the placental barrier and affect the child by blocking the deleterious effects of the immunopathologic antibodies or by causing direct damage in the fetus.

D. Galmarini et al. (eds.), Drugs and the Liver: High Risk Patients and Transplantation, 61–66.

DIAPLACENTAL PASSAGE

Like all biologic membranes, the placenta is permeable to lipophilic substances (1). The passage of hydrophilic molecules takes place via water-filled pores, thus making a detour around the lipid barrier; the placenta has such a high proportion of pores that hydrophilic substances can pass almost as fast as hydrophobic substances.

The diaplacental exchange can be considered an active function. For all practical purposes, every substance can pass from the mother to the fetus, unless it is changed or destroyed. The placenta should be regarded as a metabolically active organ that has several enzyme systems. We could also consider the placenta as a complement to the fetal tissue, which metabolizes a great number of substances to a limited degree.

DRUG METABOLISM IN THE HUMAN FETUS

Until recently it was believed that the human fetus was protected from the more hydrophilic drugs by an effective placental-fetal barrier. Even lipophilic agents that did cross the barrier would be excreted unchanged back into maternal compartment, because drug-metabolizing enzymes were not active in the placenta or fetus.

Nevertheless now we know that most drugs cross the placental-fetal barrier and equilibrate between maternal and fetal compartments. In addition, the human fetus and placenta have been shown to possess considerable drug-metabolic activity (2). Initially inert drugs may be metabolized to intermediates with specific toxicities. It is also possible that drug metabolites, which are more polar than their parent molecules, accumulate in the fetus because of the ionic trap mechanism.

Microsomes from human fetal liver catalyze many drug-metabolic reactions; the metabolic range is wide and comparable to that of the adult liver tissue. Most authors have measured enzyme levels that are 30 to 50 percent of the adult levels, and the capacity of fetal drug metabolism is comparable to that of the adult human.

Glucuronidation is quantitatively the most important of the phase II reactions in adult liver. Glucuronidation is not well developed in human fetal liver. Other conjugation reactions, however, show activities very close to those seen in adult liver.

PREDNISONE

Prednisone is a drug with relatively low-risk in pregnancy, and is used in almost all protocols for organ transplant patient. The greatest risks from corticosteroids for the pregnant patient are chronic suppression of adrenal secretions and need for boost therapy at the time of delivery (3). The stress of labor, caesarean section, or both, dictate an increase in dosage.

Several reports suggested an association between prednisone or prednisolone and malformation; however, this suspicion has not been confirmed in larger, more controlled studies.

Animal studies demonstrated an increase in fetal cleft palate following maternal ingestion of high corticosteroid doses. With doses used in clinical practice, however, the risk appears to be low. In analysis of several hundred cases reported in the literature the incidence of cleft palate in exposed children was slightly higher than in a random sample (4). Was found no evidence of a teratogenic effect for corticosteroids when comparing the maternal drug histories of the mothers of 764 infants born with anomalies of the C.N.S. and 764 controls, and no striking differences in birth weight and frequency of small for dates infants born to mothers who received systemic corticosteroids during pregnancy and those who did not (5).

Investigators also have reported intrauterine growth retardation (IUGR). However, IUGR may results from an underlying pathology rather than from the medication alone.

The amount of prednisone crossing the placenta is smaller than the amount present in maternal circulation because it is converted to prednisolone. There is only minimal risk of suppression of adrenal secretion in the fetus.

Similarly, congenital citomegalovirus infection was reported in the infant of a woman receiving azathioprine and prednisone for renal transplantation.

AZATHIOPRINE

Azathioprine is associated with an increased risk of infection and neoplasia for the pregnant patient. The increased infection-risk may be particularly significant for its potential impact on the fetus.

In addition, liver toxicity is known to occur with azathioprine and this effect may be potentiated in pregnancy. Bone-marrow depression has also been reported, but it is probably not enhanced by pregnancy.

Azathioprine can cross the placenta, and its primary metabolite, mercaptopurine, has been found in cord blood. Scattered reports have not noted malformation associated with the use of azathioprine. From a detailed analysis of successful pregnancies notified to the European Dialysis and Transplant Association, only 7 of 110 babies born to 97 women with renal transplants had congenital anomalies, one of them being a congenital citomegalovirus infection. Abnormalities were trivial in 3 babies. Chromatid breaks were found in 2 of 16 babies who unterwent chromosome analysis. Mothers of the 7 babies with abnormalities had taken significantly high daily doses of azathioprine compared with those who had normal babies. This congenital abnormality-rate is probably not excessive if we compare with a reported figure of 2% for all births (6).

Investigators have also found immunosuppression in newborns, as well as intrauterine growth retardation and bone-marrow suppression.

However, the data regarding azathioprine use in pregnancy overall appear favorable and fetal risks are far outweighed by the benefit of preserving allograft function.

CYCLOSPORINE

Cyclosporine targets T-lymphocytes without depressing bone marrow or leukocyte counts, that's why it carries less risk of infection and neoplasia. However, cyclosporine is associated with nephrotoxicity and hepatotoxicity. Cyclosporine is reported to cross the placenta and to be distributed into breast milk. However, there is an increased risk of immunosuppression in the fetus, and possibly an increased risk of fetal exposure to viral infections and subsequently congenital viral syndromes.

The blocking effect of cyclosporine on the release by helper T-lymphocytes of interleukin-2 might interfere with the differentiation of osteoclasts and osteoblasts from the stem cell. In this way, the drug could induce bone defects.

Have been reported on 6 pregnancies in renal transplant patients receiving Cyclosporine and cortisone; 2 of 6 babies were growth-retarded (7).

CYCLOPHOSPHAMIDE

Cyclophosphamide is no longer routinely used in many transplant protocol. It primarily suppresses leukocyte production and function and inhibits a broad nonspecific range of enzymatic activities that produces several side effects, including opportunistic infection, neoplasia, marrow depression, and gonadal suppression. Many men and women who take this drug display suboptimal fertility.

Cyclophosphamide is a known fetal teratogen (8). Many have reported a broad range of malformations with fetal exposure, as well as fetal bone-marrow suppression, IUGR, and possible gonadal suppression (9).

To avoid malformations and an increased risk of long-term effects, do not give cyclophosphamide during pregnancy. Transplant patients should be switched to less toxic medications well before they attempt conception.

METHOTREXATE

Methotrexate was used in organ transplant therapy several years ago, it is still given during or after bone-marrow transplants. However, it is seldom administered now for chronic maintenance.

Methotrexate, have many teratogenic effects, and has been used as an abortifacient. The range of specific malformations associated with methotrexate and with aminopterin, another folic-acid antagonist, include cranial anomalies, cleft lip and palate, low-set ears, neural tube defects, and skeletal abnormalities (10). This set of malformations does not occur in all exposed infants, and it less likely to appear in infants who were exposed during the second and third trimesters. However, second and third-trimester exposure involves an increased risk of bone- marrow suppression and possible abnormal neurologic development.

The pregnant transplant patient should not be given methotrexate and the patient considering pregnancy should be switched to an alternative therapy well before she attempts conception.

NON SPECIFIC LYMPHOCYTE ANTIBODY PREPARATIONS

Antilymphocyte and antithymocyte globulins have been used to reduce rejection reactions in transplant patients. Both globulins contain large quantities of extraneous antibodies that suppress lymphocytes and leukocytes but also cause troublesome effects. Today they are not used frequently because of problems arising from their extraneous antibodies. Purifying them is difficult and is lessened the effectiveness of treatment.

Patients treated with these immunoglobulins may have toxic reactions and occasionally experience serum sickness. They also appear to be at increased risk for infection and lymphomas (11). The effects of antilymphocyte and antithymocyte globulins in the developing fetus are unknown. The IgG component of these globulins can cross the placenta, and may have an unfavorable long-term effect on lymphocyte production or function. Moreover, the long-term impact of fetal exposure, even to these drugs, is not known.

As all immunosuppressive agents affect the immune system and T-lymphocyte production, we cannot say that in-utero exposure to any of them is free of risk. Usually, a combination of agents is needed to prevent organ rejection. Substantial experience with prednisone and azathioprine suggests that these drugs are well tolerated by the fetus. Cyclosporine may also prove fairly safe, although data are relatively scanty.

REFERENCES

1- ONNIS A., GRELLA P. (1984) The biochemical effects of drugs in pregnancy. Ellis Horwood, Chichester.
2- GRELLA P.V. (1992): In: Terapie farmacologiche materne e fetali, edited by G.B. Candiani, V. Danesino and A. Gastaldi pp. 147-160. Masson, Milano.
3- FRASER F.C., FAINSTAT T.D. (1951) Pediatrics, 8: 527-530.
4- POPERT A.J. (1962) Br. Med. J., 1: 967.
5- WARRELL D.W., TAYLOR R. (1968) Lancet, i: 117.
6- The Registration Committee of the European Dialysis and

Transplant Association (1980) Brit. J. Obstet. Gynaecol., 87: 839-845.

7- NIESERT S., GUNTER H., FREI U. (1988) Brit. Med. J., 296: 1736-1740.

8- ROUBENOFF R., HOYT J., PETRI M. (1988) Seminars in Arthritis and Rheumatism, 18: 88-90.

9- KUMAR R., BIGGART J.D., McEVOY J. (1972) Lancet, i: 1212- 1213.

10- SHAW E.B., REES E.L.(1980) Am. J. Dis. Child., 134: 1172-1178.

11- Monoclonal Antibodies for kidney allograft rejection (1986) Med. Letter, 28: 97.

REPRODUCTION AFTER TRANSPLANTATION

V. Scantlebury and T.E. Starzl

The success of orthotopic liver transplantation (OLTx) has greatly improved since the introduction of cyclosporine in 1980. Many young patients are given a second chance at life, and with this comes the restoration of menstrual abnormalities and the possibility of pregnancy [1, 2]. Since the first successful pregnancy in a liver transplant patient took place in 1976 [3, 4], a total of 29 babies have been born to 22 liver transplant recipients from the combined programs of the University of Colorado and the University of Pittsburgh. The complications and outcome of these pregnancies are reviewed and the effect on hepatic function is analyzed.

Background

Four patients underwent OLTx at the University of Colorado prior to 1980, while 18 patients received their liver transplantations at the University of Pittsburgh between 1983 and 1990. The indications for transplantation consisted primarily of chronic active hepatitis (10 patients) and fulminant hepatitis (3 patients). Two were transplanted for alpha-1 antitrypsin deficiency and sclerosing cholangitis, while biliary atresia, Wilson's disease, Caroli's disease, primary biliary cirrhosis, secondary biliary cirrhosis and Budd-Chiari Syndrome were the indications in one case each. Immunosuppression consisted of combinations of prednisone, azathioprine and/or cyclosporine in all but one patient who received the new immunosuppressive drug FK506 and prednisone. Two patients were switched from cyclosporine to FK506 1.2 and 6.5 years later.

One patient was transplanted acutely for fulminant hepatic failure during pregnancy, presenting at 26 weeks gestation [5]. All others conceived between 3 weeks and 11 1/2 years after transplantation (Table 1).

D. Galmarini et al. (eds.), Drugs and the Liver: High Risk Patients and Transplantation, 67–72.

TABLE I

CONCEPTION TIME AFTER TRANSPLANTATION

	NO. OF PATIENTS
WITHIN FIRST YEAR	11*
0-6 MONTHS	3*
6-12 MONTHS	7
WITHIN 1 TO 3 YEARS	7
AFTER 3 YEARS	5

* One patient was 26 weeks pregnant at transplantation

The patient who received FK506 and prednisone immediately after OLTx became pregnant within 15 months, but underwent an elective termination of pregnancy. This patient did not deliver any children after OLTx and therefore was not included in this study. Four other abortions after OLTx were reported: two patients each had a spontaneous abortion prior to successfully completing a pregnancy; one other had 2 therapeutic abortions after a difficult pre-term delivery.

Results

Twenty-two recipients of orthotopic liver transplantation delivered 29 children, including 2 sets of twins. Five patients each had 2 successful pregnancies. Eleven babies were born by normal spontaneous vaginal deliver (NSVD), 8 of which were full term babies; three were preterm (27%), delivered before 36 weeks gestational age. Mean birth weight in this group was 2660 grams. Fourteen of the remaining 16 deliveries performed by cesarean section resulted in preterm infants (88%), with a mean gestational age of 32 weeks. The average birth weight for cesarean births was 1820 grams. Preeclampsia was seen in 5 patients, and was the cause of early delivery in 4 of these (3 by cesarean, 1 by NSVD). Premature rupture of membranes and fetal distress were also included as frequent causes of cesarean deliveries (3 each). Other less frequent precipitating factors were breech presentation (1), transverse lie (1), intrauterine growth retardation (1) and previous cesarean delivery (4).

One repeated antepartum maternal complication seen was anemia, demonstrated in six patients (hemoglobin less than 10g/lb). Two patients were anemic from their first prenatal visit, and required red blood cell transfusions during and after their pregnancies. Progressive hypertension was seen in 2 patients, while recurrent urinary tract infection and pyelonephritis complicated the courses of 2 additional patients.

The alterations in hepatic enzyme function seen in patients are summarized as seen in Table 2. Two patients had biopsy proven rejection in the first and third trimester of pregnancy. The first one underwent treatment with steroids for presumed acute rejection, a diagnosis later changed to chronic rejection. This patient continued to have elevated transaminase enzymes throughout pregnancy. The second patient was diagnosed with acute rejection in the third trimester, biopsy also showing areas consistent with a hepatitic process. Treatment was withheld until after deliver, with near resolution of the abnormal transminases even before steroid therapy was initiated. A third biopsy performed in a patient with hepatitis B, was consistent with mild hepatitis in the second trimester of pregnancy. Four other patients had transaminase enzyme elevations in the antepartum period, and without treatment, resolved spontaneously in the immediate post-partum period. There were no reported changes in hepatic graft function in the remaining fifteen patients.

Progressive increase in hepatic enzyme activity occurred in ten patients in the post-partum period, half of whom had stable hepatic function prior to delivery. Four patients were treated empirically with steroids, while four others underwent a liver biopsy and/or percutaneous transhepatic cholangiogram (PTC).

TABLE II

ALTERATIONS IN LIVER FUNCTIONS

ANTEPARTUM	
STABLE FUNCTION	15
ENZYME ELEVATIONS	7
BIOPSY	3
POST PARTUM	
STABLE	12
ENZYME ELEVATIONS	10
STEROID TREATMENT	4
BIOPSY AND/OR PTC*	4
SPONTANEOUS RESOLUTION	3

*PTC: Percutaneous Transhepatic Cholangiogram

Two patients who had biopsies and PTC's had normal results; one was found to have ongoing hepatitis by biopsy. The fourth patient underwent a PTC after no improvement was seen with steroid treatment, and was found to have multiple biliary structures by cholangiogram. This patient had chronic rejection diagnosed in the first trimester, and underwent re-transplantation within 2 months after delivery.

Of the twenty-nine infants born to women who received liver transplantation, one was conceived 27 weeks prior to an emergency OLTx for fulminant hepatic B. A second OLTx was required on post-op day 3 due to primary graft failure. As a result of multiple complications, a cesarean delivery was carried out 1 week later, with subsequent death of the neonate. Of the remaining 28 babies conceived after transplantation, a second death occurred in an infant born at 26 weeks gestation, whose mother developed severe preeclampsia. This child died from presumed sepsis after becoming neutropenic (5). A third death occurred in a 7 month old infant born to a patient 10 years after her transplant and 3 1/2 years after the birth of her first child (6). A diagnosis for the human immunodeficiency virus infection was made in both mother and child, both of whom later succumbed to the complications of this virus infection. One other maternal death was reported in a 25 year old mother who developed B-cell lymphoma 2 1/2 years after the birth of her child (7).

Other neonatal complications reported include intrauterine growth retardation (4) hyperbilirubinemia (4), respiratory insufficiency requiring ventilatory assistance in 2 patients, retrolental hyperplasia and methadone withdrawal in one patient each. All children are said to be developing normally and no congenital abnormalities were reported.

Discussion

Transplantation has evolved as an accepted procedure for failed organs, but the long term effects of immunosuppression still remain a concern. Previous publications regarding pregnancy following renal transplantation [8 - 10], have reported complications such as congenital abnormalities, adrenocortical insufficiency, infections, liver dysfunction and seizures. These patients were immunosuppressed with azathioprine and steroids, at dosages higher than those used today. Only four patients received azathioprine as the main immunosuppressive agent. Although there were neonatal complications reported in one child [6], no long term sequelae were observed.

Cyclosporine has been shown to cross the placenta [11], and levels have been reported in the newborns born to mothers on CyA. Our report documents the use of this immunosuppressive agent in 18 patients who received liver transplantation without any significant adverse sequelae. FK506, the newest immunosuppressive agent was used in 3 patients, 2 of whom delivered babies. Both of these had a history of CyA use and received FK506 only for 2 weeks and 8 months prior to pregnancy. No valid conclusion can be drawn from the use of this agent in such short intervals of time.

The risk of rejection does not appear to be increased during pregnancy, with only one case of acute rejection diagnosed by biopsy. Despite enzyme elevations seen, those not treated immediately underwent resolution along with those that received treatment. 30% of the patients had increasing hepatic enzyme activity in the antepartum period with 45% having alterations in the post-partum period. Again, spontaneous resolution occurred in 50% of cases.

Overall, of 29 babies born to 22 liver transplant recipients, 60% of births occurred by cesarean delivery with a 88% incidence of prematurity seen in this group. Contributing factors were prelampsia, premature rupture of membranes, and early fetal distress. Neonates born by NSVD sustained less maternal complications and were more normal in size, while 10% of babies delivered at full gestational age were small for gestational age. No congenital abnormalities were reported, and except for 3 infant deaths (10%), all others are reported to be alive and well. It is reasonable to assume that liver transplant recipients can still undergo a successful pregnancy, but it is not without risks. We suggest that careful monitoring be carried out by both a perinatologist and a transplant physician in order to minimize complications to both mother and child.

REFERENCES

1. de Koning N.D., Haagsma E.B. (1990):Digestion 46: 239-241.
2. Cundy T.F., O'Grady J.G., Williams R. (1990):Gut 31:337-338.
3. Myers R.L., Schmid R, Newton J.J. (1980):Transplantation 29:432.
4. Walcott W.O., Derick D.E., Jolley J.J., Snyder D.L. (1978):Am J. Obstet and Gynecol 132:340-341.
5. Laifer S.A., Darby M.J., Scantelbury V.P., Harger J.H., Caritis S.N. (1990):Obstet Gynecol 76:1083-1088.
6. Newton E.R., Turksoy N., Kaplan M., Reinhold R. (1988):Obstet Gynecol 71:499-500.
7. Scantlebury V., Gordon R., Tzakis A., Koneru B., Bowman J., Mazzaferro V., Stevenson W.C., Todo S., Iwatsuki I., Starzl T.E. (1990):Transplantation 49:317-321.
8. Penn I. and Makowski E.L. (1981):Transplantation Proc. 13:36-39.
9. Penn I., Makowski E.L., Harris P. (1980): Transplantation 30:397-400.
10. Scott J.R. (1977):Am. J. Obstet Gynecol 128:668-674.
11. Vankataramanan R., Koneru B., Wang C.C., Burckart G.J., Caritis S.N., Starzl T.E. (1988): Transplantation 46:468-469.

REPRODUCTION IN HBsAg+ LIVER RECIPIENTS

REPRODUCTION AFTER LIVER TRANSPLANTATION FOR B-VIRUS HEPATITIS

G.Rossi, L.R.Fassati, B.Gridelli, M.Colledan, U.Maggi, P.Reggiani, G.Paone, L.Caccamo, A.Lucianetti, S.Gatti, A.Piazzini, M.Doglia and D.Galmarini

INTRODUCTION

Larger and larger population of patients are coming to liver transplantation and the reproductive potential of these patients is of significant concern to those involved.

Clinical experience with renal transplantation and subsequent reproduction has demonstrated the possibility and safety of pregnancy after liver transplantation.

The first successful pregnancy in a liver transplant recipient took place in 1976 (1). Isolated cases of pregnancy are reported (2-3-4-5-6-7-8-9-10-11) until 1990 when a large series of 20 infants born to 17 liver transplant recipients was published (12); at present this last series reached 29 infants (Scantlebury personal comunication). Much more has been written about pregnancy after renal transplantation (3).

In 1981 Penn (3) reported that 50 male renal transplants have been responsible of 67 pregnancies under azathioprine but no male liver transplant recipients have fathered any children. Eleven paternities from male patients on cyclosporine therapy were reported in 1989 (13).

Orthotopic liver transplantation (OLTx) is not a contraindication to bearing children despite the increased risk to the mother (e.g. hypertension, anemia, elevation of liver enzymes, increased number of caesarian births) and to the fetus (e.g. prematurity, intrauterine growth retardation) as compared to

D. Galmarini et al. (eds.), Drugs and the Liver: High Risk Patients and Transplantation, 73–78.

the normal population (12).

When OLTx is performed in patients HBsAg positive a further risk for mother and fetus is added. Hepatitis B virus (HBV) in fact could influence both mother and child and active/passive immunoprophylaxis is requireds to prevent graft reinfection and infection of the fetus.

Infants born to women who are positive for hepatitis-B-surface antigen are at risk for development of acute liver disease, chronic liver disease and hepatocellular carcinoma and act as community reservoirs for the virus (14-15).

Without HBV immunoprophylaxis in infants born to HBsAg carrier mothers perinatal HBV infection rates range from 10% to 90% depending from the virological status of the mother; with active/passive immunoprophylaxis in the newborn infection rate decreases to 1%-10% (14-16-17-18-19).

MATERIALS AND METHODS

Out of 137 OLTx performed in 121 patients 42 were female in childbearing age and 3 became pregnant 26-42 months after the transplant (OLTx: 7-8-42) but one of these (OLTx 42) ended in voluntary abortion as parenthood was not desired.

Mean age at time of pregnancy was 23 years. All 3 patients were HBsAg positive at the time of OLTx for post-hepatitic cirrhosis (OLTx 7-8) and for fulminant hepatitis (OLTx 42).

Two children were also conceived from fathers 28-14 months after OLTx performed for HBsAg positive cirrhosis (OLTx 18-72).

All these patients were treated with active/passive immunoprophylaxis against HBV. The last protocol that we are using in all patients transplanted for HBsAg positive hepatopathy consists of:

- active immunization with 50 mcg of HBV-DNA recombinant vaccination during the anhepatic phase at 1-2-12 months;
- passive immunization starts during the anhepatic phase with 10.000 I.U. of i.v. hyperimmune anti HBV immunoglobulines (HBIg): a protective titre of HBsAb is maintained with i.m. administration of HBIg (600 I.U. for 6 months; 200 I.U. thereafter) (20).

All patients (female and male) were HBsAg negative at the time of conceiving.

Immunosuppression was maintained with cyclosporine A (CsA) (OLTx 8), steroids + azathioprine (AZA)(OLTx 7) and steroids + CsA (OLTx 18-72 male patients).

Gynecological history in OLTx 8 was characterized by difficulty in maintaining pregnancies before and after OLTx with 4 spontaneous abortion and a premature birth with death of the child and secondary amenorrhoea before OLTx; two months after OLTx menstruation recovered and 2 abortions occured before having a successful pregnancy 3 years and 8 months after OLTx.

In OLTx 7 there was primary amenorrhoea with spontaneous recovery of menstruation 4 months after OLTx and successful pregnancy 3 years and 9 months after OLTx.

About pregnancy management all recipients were classified as high-risk patients and closely managed by both obstetricians and transplant surgeons.

At birth we have used the same active/passive immunoprophylaxis against HBV, like for infants born to mothers HBsAg positive, and consists of i.m. HBIg at birth (0,5 ml/Kg - 1 ml = 90 I.U.) and 20 mcg of HBV-DNA recombinant vaccination at birth, 1 and 6 months.

RESULTS

Both patients (OLTx 8-7) demonstrated, during the third trimester, moderate increase in transaminases (GOT-GPT), gamma-GT, alkaline phosphatase, bilirubin conditioning 2 caesarian sections (C.S.).

The child born from OLTx 8 (Immunosuppression = CsA) was premature (32 weeks) and C.S. was perfomed after establishing pulmonary maturity; the newborn weighted 2190 grams with an APGAR score of 7 and 8 at the first and fifth minute without congenital abnormalities.

A term child (37 weeks), weighing 4260 grams, was born from OLTx 7 (Immunosuppression = AZA + steroids) with an APGAR score of 7 and 9 at the first and fifth minute; ecocardiography, performed without any clinical indication, showed patency of interatrial foramen ovalae and of Botallo's duct but both defects disappeared spontaneously in few days.

Both children at birth were HBsAg negative and were treated with the previous described protocol of active/passive immunoprophylaxis against HBV and, at present, are HBsAg negative and HBsAb positive rispectively 24 and 14 months after delivery with normal development.

Both children were fed artificially just to prevent ingetions of CsA or AZA with mother's milk.

Milk's CsA levels, tested in OLTx 8, were in fact always higher than in blood.

The abnormalities of hepatic function, during the third trimester of pregnancy, were not consistent with rejection and resoled spontaneously.

No infant had complications as a results of exposure to chronic immunosuppression.

Two children were also conceived from fathers on CsA-steroids medication after a liver transplant (OLTx 18-72) performed for post-hepatitic HBsAg positive cirrhosis; these children were conceived with women HBsAg negative.

DISCUSSION

The infant born to mother on AZA+steroids was on term and with normal weight while the infant born to mother on CsA was premature and small for gestational age. Prematurity and intrauterine growth retardation seem a major problem with CsA than with AZA and some authors suggest to use rather AZA + steroids in future pregnancies of transplanted patients also if further observations are necessary (9-21-22-23).

Two healthy children were also conceived from transplanted fathers under CsA medication despite the testicular disfunction with sterility or reduction of fertility described in animals treated with CsA (24).

No congenital anomalies were observed with the exception of a transitory asymptomatic patency of Botallo's duct and interatrial foramen.

Subsequent alternations in their reproductive capacity, later in adulthood, has yet to be evalutated.

CsA and AZA are expressed in the breast milk and patients should be advised not to breast feed (13). Breast feeding is also considered an important factor in vertical transmission of HBV from mother to newborn.

In transplanted patients there is an increased incidence of complications in mothers and babies which apparently results from organ transplantation. Therefore female wishing to conceive should be informed of these risks and we advise not to become pregnant those with impaired hepatic, renal function and difficult control of hypertension (5-13).

At conceiving all our patients were HBsAg negatve but infants were treated as if born to mothers HBsAg positive. In fact the most part of HBsAg+ patients transplanted and treated with active/passive HBV immunooprophylaxis, did not elicit in active seroconversion and the titre of HBsAb was maintained owing to i.m. administration of HBIg.

In these patients if HBIg are withdrawn HBV recurrence is almost sure suggesting that, despite HBsAg negativity in blood, HBV is prenset in some body reservoir.

HBIg act as a protective barrier for the new liver but are not successful in clearing completely HBV from the body and so we have to consider these patients like HBsAg positive.

Despite the increased risk for mother and newborn pregnancy is not contraindicated also in patients transplanted for HBsAg positive hepatopathy if a correct protocol of active/passive immunoprophylaxis against HBV is followed.

REFERENCES

1) Walcott W.O., Derick D.E., Jolley J.J. and Snyder D.L. (1978): Am. J. Obstet. Gyenecol., 132:340-341.
2) Myers R.L., Schmid R. and Newton J.J. (1980): Transplantation, 29:432-435.
3) Penn I., Makowski E.L. (1981): Transplant. Proc., 13:36-39.
4) Newton E.R., Turksoy N., Kaplan M. and Reinhold R. (1988): Obstet. Gynecol., 71:499-500.
5) Venkataramanan R., Koneru B., Wang C.C., Burckart G.J., Caritis S. and Starzl T.E. (1988): Transplantation, 46:468-469.
6) Sims C.J., Porter K.B. and Knuppel R.A. (1989): Am. J. Obstet. Gynecol., 161:532-533.
7) Haagsma E.B., Visser G.H., Klompmaker I.J., Verwer R. and Slooff M.J. (1989): Obstet. Gynecol., 74:442-443.
8) Alvin P., Muller J., Houssin D., Pras-Jude N., Chapuis Y. and Courtecuisse V. (1989): Gastroenterol. Clin. Biol., 13:1079-1081.
9) Cundy T.F., O'Grady J.G. and Williams R. (1990): Gut, 31:337-338.
10) Bourget P., Fernandez H., Bismuth H. and Papiernik E. (1990): Transplantation, 49:663.
11) Kreuzpaintner G., Ringe B., Niesert S., Pichlmayr R. and Strohmeyer G. (1990): Dtsch. Med. Wochenscher, 115:895-898.
12) Scantlebury V., Gordon R., Tzakis A., Koneru B., Bowman J., Mazzaferro V., Stevenson W.C., Todo S., Iwatsuki S. and Starzl T.E. (1990): Transplantation, 49:317-321.

13) Cockburn I., Krupp P. and Monka C. (1989): Transplant. Proc., 21:3730-3732.
14) Jonas M.M., Reddy R.K., Medina M. and Schiff E.R. (1990): Am. J. Gastroenterol., 85:277-280.
15) Phuapradit P. and Varavithya W. (1989): J. Med. Assoc. Thai., 72(s):84-87.
16) Henrietta M.H., Lelie P.N., Wong V.C.W., Kuhns M.C. and Reesink H.W. (1989): Lancet, i:406-409.
17) Schalm S.W. and Pit-Grosheide P. (1989): Lancet, i:44.
18) Schermann D.J.C. and Finlayson N.D.C. (1989): In "Disease of the gastrointestinal tract and liver", edited by D.J.C. Shermannn and N.D.C. Finlayson pp. 970-971. Churchill Livingstone, Edinburgh.
19) Shi-Xin-Tang and Guang-Lieh Yu. (1990): Lancet, i:302.
20) Colledan M., Grendele M., Gridelli B., Rossi G., Fassati L.R., Ferla G., Doglia M., Gislon M. and Galmarini D. (1989): Transplant. Proc., 21:2421-2423.
21) Niesert S. and Günter H. (1988): Brit. Med. J., 296:1736.
22) Al-Khader A.A., Absy M., Al-Hasani, Joyce B. and Sabbagh T. (1988): Transplantation, 45:987-988.
23) Pickrell M.D. and Michael J. (1988): Brit. Med. J., 296:825.
24) Seethalakshmi L., Diamond D.A.,Malhotra R.K., Mazanitis S.G., Kumar S. and Menon M. (1988): Transplant. Proc., 20:1005-1010.

24 HOUR-HYPOTHERMIC PRESERVATION OF RAT LIVER WITH EURO-COLLINS AND UW SOLUTIONS. COMPARATIVE EVALUATION BY 31P NMR SPECTROSCOPY, BIOCHEMICAL ASSAYS AND LIGHT MICROSCOPY.

J-M. GULIAN , C. DALMASSO , S. MASSON , F. DESMOULIN ,
C. SCHEINER , M. CHARREL and P.J. COZZONE .

INTRODUCTION

Advances in liver preservation had been slow, until Jamieson et al. (1) described a successful long-term cold-preservation of the dog liver based on the use of a lactobionate-containing solution. However, additional progress has remained limited for two reasons. First, the mechanisms responsible for cellular injury induced by cold-ischemic preservation are not fully understood due to the complexity of events occurring during storage and reperfusion. Second, the evaluation of the metabolic status of the transplant during ischemia and reperfusion has lacked adequate invasive and non-invasive methodologies.

Liver viability after cold ischemic preservation, may be investigated in animal models by a variety of methods: survival time after organ transplantation, histological studies of cell viability or morphological appearance by light or electron microscopy, chemical determinations on tissue extracts, liver effluents and preservation solutions, and analysis by NMR, *in vivo* or on excised organs. The results obtained by these methods are complementary and need to be correlated since they reflect various aspects of cellular metabolism function and morphology.

In this paper, we report a comparative study of 24 hr preservation at 4°C of excised rat liver using Euro-Collins (EC) and University of Wisconsin (UW) solutions. The quality of preservation has been assessed based on (i) the cellular energy status determined non invasively by 31P NMR spectroscopy and (ii) the extent of cellular injury estimated from the loss of purine compounds during ischemia and reperfusion measured by HPLC, the leakage of intracellular enzymes and the modifications of parenchyma established by light microscopy.

MATERIALS AND METHODS

Preservation solutions

EC solutions were prepared by the Central Pharmacy of the Hopital de la Timone (Marseille, France). The UWm was prepared in the laboratory and did not contain hydroxy-ethyl starch.

D. Galmarini et al. (eds.), Drugs and the Liver: High Risk Patients and Transplantation, 79–84.

Liver preparation

Male rats of the Wistar strain (body weight 246±8 g) were used as liver donors. In order to ensure controlled and reproducible metabolic conditions, the animals were submitted to a 24 hr-fast followed by a meal 8 hr prior to liver excision. Rats livers were prepared and perfused as described by Desmoulin et al. (2).

Preservation protocol

The preservation protocols included three steps: a 40 min-control period at 20°C, followed by 24 hr of ischemia at 2-4°C and 30 min of reperfusion at 20°C. The liver was perfused with a Krebs-Heinseleit (KH) medium during the control period while three NMR spectra were recorded. At the end of this equilibration period, a liver fragment was cut off for light microscopy and the liver was rinsed with 100 ml of ice cooled/N2 gassed EC or UWm solutions. Then, the liver was transferred in a small plastic bag containing 54±3.2 ml of the preservation solution and stored at 2-4°C. After 24 hr of ischemia, a volume of 54±3.9 ml of the effluent perfusate (reperfusion medium) was collected during the first 1.8±0.13 min of reperfusion with oxygenated KH at 20°C. An aliquot of the storage medium where the liver had been bathing for the 24 hr was taken. The samples of the storage medium and the effluent were stored at -80°C for subsequent biochemical analyses. Before introducing the reperfused liver in the NMR tube, another biopsy was taken. Spectra were recorded at 8 and 30 min after the onset of reperfusion.

NMR experiments

31P NMR experiments were carried out on a Nicolet NT200-WB spectrometer at 80.9 MHz without proton decoupling as already described (2) using a 30 mm diameter NMR cell. For quantification, areas were corrected for differential saturation effects (2).

Biochemical assays

Potassium, lactate dehydrogenase (LDH) and AST activities were determined by conventional procedures using an automatic analyzer (Hitachi 717). Compounds of the purine nucleotides catabolism including inosine, hypoxanthine, xanthine and uric acid were assayed by HPLC with UV detection as already described (3).

Light microscopy

The hepatic biopsies were immediately fixed in 10% formalin andembedded in paraffin. Sections of 4 micron- thickness were stained with hematoxylin and eosin.

Data analysis

Data are presented as means ± SEM, with the number of observations in parenthesis. Statistical analysis between experimental groups were performed using the unpaired, two tailed Student's t-test. A p value less than 0.05 was considered as significant.

RESULTS

NMR spectroscopy

A typical 31P NMR spectrum, characteristic of a well-perfused rat liver, is presented in figure 1A. It shows a high NTP content and a low inorganic phosphate (Pi) level (NTP/Pi=1.63±0.17; n=13). The intracellular pH is 7.24±O.O5 (n=13).

A Control spectrum

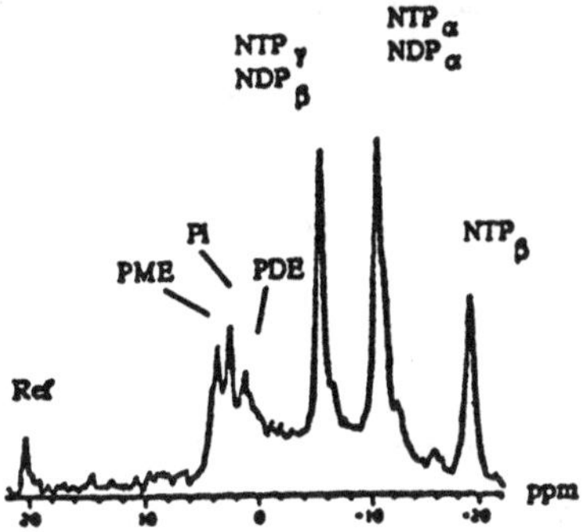

B Spectra after 30 min of reperfusion

after 24 hr storage in UWm

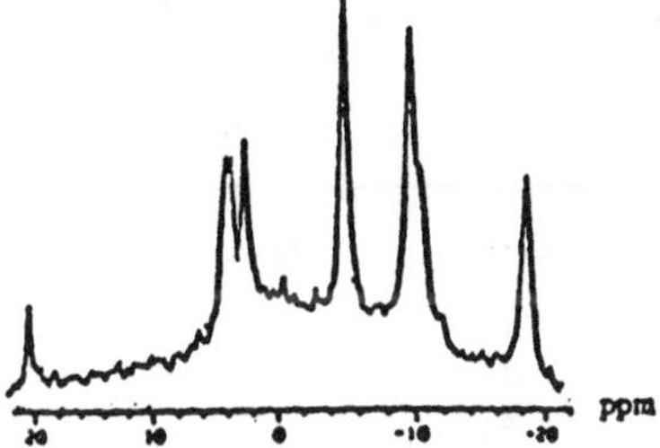

after 24 hr storage in EC

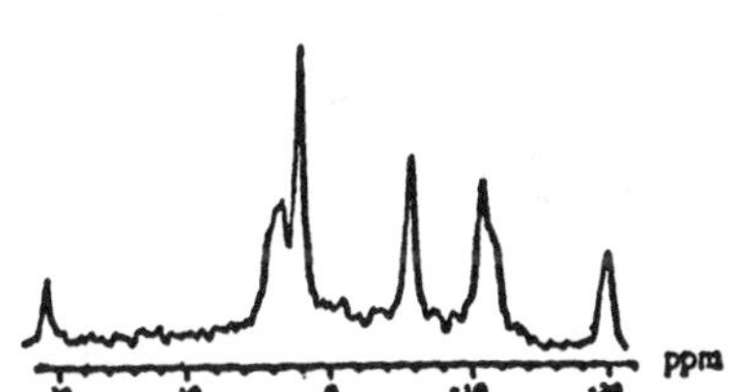

FIG.1, 31P NMR spectra of rat liver recorded at 80.9: A, before ischemia, B, after 30 min of reperfusion. Ref, hexachlorocyclotriphosphazene, at 20.65 ppm; PME, phosphomonoesters; Pi, inorganic phosphate; PDE, phosphodiesters; NTP, nucleosides 5'-triphosphate; NDP, nucleosides 5'-diphosphate.

The contribution to the intracellular Pi signal from vascular Pi can be neglected due to (i) the low Pi concentration in the KH medium (1.2 mM) and (ii) the small extracellular volume (4, 5). After 24 hours of ischemia, NMR visible NTP and NDP disappear totally. The remaining resonances mainly arise from Pi, phosphomonoesters and NAD-NADH in the diphosphodiester region. Spectra 1B have been acquired after 30 min of reperfusion. The extent of NTP recovery is respectively 58 and 80% after 8 min for the EC and UWm groups. After 30 min, NTP reached a similar plateau in the two groups. Pi levels were significantly higher in the EC group than in the UWm group, even after 30 min of reperfusion.

Biochemical assays

TABLE 1. Production of purine catabolites and enzyme activities during storage and reperfusion with EC or UWm

	Inosine	Hypoxanthine	Xanthine	Uric Acid	Sum	AST	LDH
	(μM/100 g Body Weight)					(IU/100 g Body Weight)	
Storage bath							
EC (n=5)	*	0.11±0.08	0.14±0.06	1.37±0.13	1.61±0.15 **	0.12±0.01*	0.92±0.15*
UWm (n=8)	4.25±0.76	1.22±0.17	*	*	5.47±0.91	0.12±0.01	1.25±0.16
Reperfusate							
EC (n=5)	*	0.16 ± 0.08	1.61±0.53	5.95±1.91	7.85±2.03 **	0.57±0.14**	0.13±0.03*
UWm (n=8)	0.14±0.02	0.27±0.02	*	*	0.41±0.04	0.21±0.02	0.22±0.05

* Signal intensity under the detection limit.
Comparison of storage bath and reperfusate of EC group vs UWm group: * NS; **$p < 0.007$.

Light microscopy

TABLE 2. Grades of morphological changes by light microscopy

Experiments	Control period (n =12)	EC group (n= 5)	UWm group (n= 7)
Number	Grade	Grade	Grade
1	1	2	
2	1	2	
3	1	2	
4	1	4	
5	1	2	
6	1		1
7	1		1
8	1		1
9	1		1
10	1		1
11	1		2
12	1		2

Grade 1 No damage; normal histological aspect
Grade 2 Mild alterations with alternation of clarification and eosinophilic condensations; ballooning of hepatocytes; normal nuclei
Grade 3 Hepatocyte microvacuolisation
Grade 4 Pyknosis of hepatocytes nuclei and cytoplasmic condensations; degenerative parenchymal changes up to cellular necrosis

DISCUSSION

After 8 min of reperfusion, NTP was maximum and stable while a decrease in Pi level was observed reaching at 30 min, values 30% (EC group) and 26% (UWm group) lower than at 8 min. This decrease suggests a net Pi efflux from the intracellular to the intravascular space which may be generated by the strong concentration gradient which prevails during reperfusion (6) or could involved the $Na^+/H_2PO_4^-$ cotransport (7,8). Transient NMR invisibility (2,9,10) or intracellular wash out (11) could also account for the Pi signal decrease. However, the stability of intracellular potassium concentration (data not shown) rules out the occurrence of the latter possible mechanism.

The higher NTP recovery observed for UWm preservation corresponds to the lower release of total purine catabolites during reperfusion. The enhanced preservation of the pool of purine compounds is due to the presence of allopurinol (1 mM) and adenosine in the UWm solution (Table 1). The efficacy of the inhibitory effect of allopurinol persists during the first minutes of reperfusion as demonstrated by the lack of xanthine and uric acid in the reperfusion effluent. The remaining intracellular concentration of allopurinol is then sufficient to achieve the inhibition of xanthine oxidase. The high concentration of inosine and hypoxanthine in the storage medium of UWm group illustrates the active catabolism of adenosine in the organ even at 4°C during the storage period. The catabolism of purine compounds goes as far as uric acid when preservation is carried out with the EC solution. The increase of the total purine catabolites during reperfusion, mainly due to xanthine and uric acid, reflects a production rather than a washout of compounds.

The leakage of AST during cold ischemia is independent from the preservation solution, suggesting that cell injury is similar in both groups (Table 1). The release of AST increases more with the duration of reperfusion in the EC group suggesting the involvement of oxygen-derived free radicals in the generation of cellular damage (12-16). During reperfusion, the supply of oxygen to reactions catalyzed by xanthine oxidase (17-23) enhances the formation of uric acid. In the EC group, high concentrations of xanthine and uric acid are found in the storage bath and the reperfusate, and AST leakage is higher, indicating that deleterious oxidative processes are operative (the EC solution is devoid of allopurinol and glutathione). Conversely, in the UWm group where xanthine oxidase is inhibited, xanthine and uric acid are not detected and the AST leakage is reduced in the reperfusate.

Histological observations on liver biopsies are more discriminative although parenchymal cells are less sensitive to ischemia-reperfusion injuries than the sinusoidal cell lining (24-27). Hepatocytes suffer higher injury in the EC group, than in the UWm group (Table 2). Swelling of hepatocytes in the EC group could be due to the water influx related to the absence of lactobionate and raffinose (28-31).

In conclusion, our study confirms and extends further previous reports in the literature which demonstrate the overall superiority of UWm solution for rat liver preservation. The combination of non-invasive methods on the liver tissue (NMR) and on the storage medium and reperfusate (biochemical and enzymatic assays), with invasive histological studies on biopsies provides a wide evaluation of the respective merits of the two solutions. It may offer a better quantitative assessment of the protective capacity of the different solutions and protocols used in liver transplant preservation which could lead to the establishment of metabolic and histological scores.

REFERENCES

1. Jamieson N.V.,Sundberg R.,Lindell S.,Claesson K.,Moen J.,Vreugdenhil P.K., Wight D.G.D.,Southard J.H. and Belzer F.O.(1988): *Transplantation,* 46: 517-522.
2. Desmoulin F.,Cozzone P. J. and Canioni P.(1987): *Eur. J. Biochem*., 162: 151-159.
3. Wynants J. and Van Belle H.(1985): *Anal. Biochem*., 144: 258-266.

4. van Berkel T. J.C., van den Berg G.B., Nagelkerke J.F., Kruijt J.K. and Koster J.F. (1981): In: *Short-term regulation of liver metabolism*, edited by L. Hue, G. Van de Werve pp. 379-388. Elsevier/North-Holland, Amsterdam.
5. Thoma W. J. and Ugurbil K.(1987): *Biochim. Biophys. Acta*, 893: 225-231.
6. Sestoft L. B. and Kristensen L. O.(1979): *Am. J. Physiol.*, 236: C202-C210.
7. Escoubet B.,Djabali K. and Amiel C.(1989): *Am. J. Physiol.*, 256: C322-C328.
8. Bernard M.,Momomura S-I.,Spencer R.G.S.,Grossman W. and Ingwall J.S.(1990): *IXth Meeting of the Society of Magnetic Resonance in Medicine*, 800.
9. Iles R. A.,Stevens A.N.,Griffiths J.R. and Morris P.G.(1985): *Biochem. J.*, 229: 141-151.
10. Murphy E.,Gabel S.A.,Funk A. and London R.E.(1988): *Biochemistry*, 27: 526-528.
11. Vine W.,Link J.,Thomas W. J. and Ugurbil K.(1989): *NMR in Biomedicine*, 2: 19-26.
12. Chaudry I.H.(1983): *Am. J. Physiol.*, 245: R117-R134.
13. Marubayashi S.,Dohi K.,Yamada K. and Kawasaki T.(1984): *Biochim. Biophys. Acta*, 797: 1-9.
14. Bulkley G.B.(1987): *Br. J. Cancer*, 55: 66-73.
15. Metzger J.,Dore S.P. and Lauterburg B.H.(1988): *Hepatology*, 8: 580-584.
16. Farber J.L.,Chien K.R. and Mittnacht S.,Jr.(1981): *Am. J. Pathol.*, 102: 271-281.
17. McCord J.M.(1985): *N. Engl. J. Med.*, 312: 159-163.
18. Granger D.N.,Hollwarth M.E. and Parks D.A.(1986): *Acta Physiol. Scand.*, 548: 47-63.
19. Hearse D.J.,Manning A.S.,Downey J.M. and Yellon D.M.(1986): *Acta Physiol. Scand.*, 548: 65-78.
20. Pietri S.,Culcasi M. and Cozzone P. J.(1989): *Eur. J. Biochem.*, 186: 163-173.
21. Engerson T.D.,McKelvey T.G.,Rhyne D.B.,Boggio E.B.,Snyder S.J. and Jones H.P. (1987): *J. Clin. Invest.*, 79: 1564-1570..
22. McKelvey T.G.,Hollwarth M.E.,Granger D.N.,Engerson T.D.,Landler U. and Jones H.P. (1988): *Am. J. Physiol.*, 254: G753-G760.
23. Friedl H.P.,Guerra E.E.,Cramer T.,Giacherio D.,Toledo-Pereyra L.H. and Till G.O.(1990): *Transplant. Proc.*, 22: 513-515.
24. McKeown C.M.B.,Edwards V.,Phillips M. J.,Harvey P.R.C.,Petrunka C.N. and Strasberg S.M.(1988): *Transplantation*, 46: 178-191.
25. Marzi I.,Zhong Z.,Zimmermann F.A.,Lemasters J. J. and Thurman R.G. (1989): *Transplant. Proc.*, 21: 1319-1320.
26. Momii S. and Koga A.(1990): *Transplantation*, 50: 745-750.
27. Currin R.T.,Toole J.G.,Thurman R.G. and Lemasters J.J.(1990): *Transplantation*, 50: 1076-1078.
28. Belzer F.O. and Southard J.H.(1988): *Transplantation*, 45: 673-676.
29. Southard J.H.(1989): *Transplant. Proc.*, 21: 1195-1196.
30. Yu W.,Coddington D. and Bitter-Suermann H.(1990): *Transplantation*, 49: 1060-1066.
31. Azuma T.,Motoshima K.,Tsunoda T.,Tsuchiya R. and Nakasono I.(1990): *Transplant. Proc.*, 22: 498.

ATP CONTENT DURING THE ISCHEMIC PERIOD AS AN INDICATOR OF LIVER VIABILITY. A PHOSPHORUS-31 NMR STUDY

J.-L. Gallis and P. Canioni

It is widely accepted that a direct correlation exits between the successfully operative allograft function and the recovery of the energetic status (ATP content) of the liver parenchyme after the cold preservation period. Phosphorus-31 Nuclear Magnetic Resonance (^{31}P NMR) is an ideal method for non-invasive observation and monitoring of energy metabolism. In addition, the chemical shift of inorganic phosphate (Pi) is pH dependent and the position of the Pi resonance in the spectrum leads to the determination of cytosolic pH (pHi) in tissues. The main objective of this paper is to discuss (i) the NMR visibility of phosphorylated metabolites in the liver in particular during cold ischemia, (ii) the changes occuring on liver energy metabolism and pHi both during hypothermic ischemia and subsequent reperfusion, and (iii) the efficiency - based on specific NMR criteria - of various preservation media including Eurocollins (EC), Belzer UW-lactobionate (UW) and Bretschneider histidine (HTK) solutions.

It is generally assumed that only "free" metabolites, at sufficiently high concentration in the cytosol (near 1 mM), can generate NMR signals. The "NMR visible" nucleoside triphosphates (NTP) are the most easily quantified compounds from the analysis of the recorded spectra (β-phosphate resonance, Figure 1). The absolute metabolite content of the tissue is determinated by comparing the area of the resonance of interest with the area of an exogenous phosphorus-

D. Galmarini et al. (eds.), Drugs and the Liver: High Risk Patients and Transplantation, 85–90.

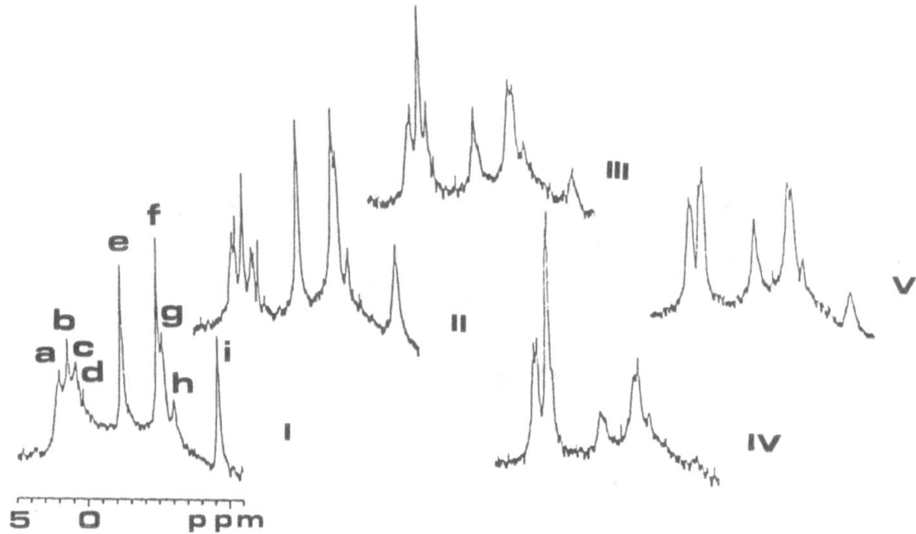

FIG.1 P-31 NMR spectra of the isolated rat liver during the sequence : perfusion - 8 hours cold ischemia - reperfusion. Typical spectra recorded during the course of the protocol are selected : liver perfused (3 ml/min/g of liver wet weight) with Krebs medium at (I) 37°C and (II) 4°C, (III) after 1 hour and (IV) after 6 hour of ischemia in Krebs medium at 4°C. Reperfusion with Krebs medium at 4°C (V) and 37°C (VI). Major resonances are assigned to (a) phosphomonoesters (PME), (b) inorganic phosphate (Pi), (c) glycerol-3-phosphorylethanolamine (GPE), (d) glycerol-3-phosphorylcholine (GPC), (e) nucleoside 5'-triphosphates (NTPγ), and -diphosphates (NDPβ), (f) NTPα and NDPα, (g) nicotinamide adenine dinucleotide (NAD & NADH), (h) uridine 5'-diphosphoglucose (UDPG), (i) NTPβ. Spectra are recorded at 161 MHz (AM400 wide-bore Bruker) in a 20 mm NMR cell; each spectrum corresponds to 240 scans (2 min accumulation), 47.5° pulse angle, 0.5 s delay between pulses.

containing compound (i.e, methylene-diphosphonic acid: MDPA) of known concentration. The NMR acquisition parameters such as the repetition rate and the flip angle are selected in order to optimize the signal to noise ratio. The optimisation depends on the longitudinal relaxation time (T_1) of the nucleus, which can varie with the temperature. Moreover, when the repetition time is lower than five fold the T_1 value, the NTP content determination must be evaluated by calculating a saturation parameter (S), from the knowledge of the flip angle, the relaxation delay and the T_1 value (1-3). Similar T_1 values were obtained for β-NTP in liver, either at 37°C or 4°C (4). This lack of temperature effect has also been observed for matrix nucleotides in isolated intact mitochondria (5).

In well oxygenated perfused liver from a fed rat, NTP are 100% NMR detectable (1-3, 6) ; an average value of 7 to 8 μmol/g liver dry weight (ca 2 to 2.5 mM for intracellular concentration) has been found for the NTP content. In agreement with these results, it has been recently demonstrated that matrix ATP is totally NMR-observable in mitochondria isolated from cold perfused liver, over a wide range of adenine nucleotide concentrations and temperature (5). In contrast, discrepancies between ATP levels measured by ^{31}P NMR on normothermic ischemic isolated liver and estimates determined by enzymic methods from perchloric acid (PCA) extracts from the same organ, suggest the existence of an NMR-invisible pool within the tissue, tentatively assigned to the mitochondrial compartment (7). The experimental approach consisting in following the relative change of tissue metabolite content with ischemia duration allows to determine whether the extent of NMR visibility of a metabolite differs with changes in cellular integrity (4). In this way, we have examined the influence of hypothermia (4°C) owing to its delaying effects on cell injury, induced by ischemic conditions (Figure 1). On the basis of their ^{31}P NMR chemical shifts, the individual purine (or pyrimidine) NTP, such as GTP, UTP, and CTP are normally indistinguishable from each other by ^{31}P NMR. In many organs (muscle, heart...), GTP, UTP, and CTP are normally present in much smaller concentrations than ATP and thus they are not thought to contribute significantly to the ^{31}P NMR spectrum. In isolated rat liver, under normoxic and normothermic perfusion, we have found by High Performance Liquid Chromatography (HPLC) analysis of PCA extracts from freeze-clamped organs, a (GTP+UTP)/ATP ratio of 0.18-0.20, in agreement with the data of others (8, 9), strongly suggesting that other NTP than ATP might contribute in a non negligible part (15-20%) to the NMR signal. Moreover, our results indicate that NTP, and thus ATP, remain fully NMR-detectable in the liver as long as the cellular integrity is maintained (Table 1). Increased mobility of paramagnetic ions, such as Mn^{++}, present in different cell compartments (mainly in mitochondria which display a Mn^{++} content of about 400 μM) could explain the partial NMR-invisibility of NTP in the liver during warm ischemia (7), and is likely to represent a manifestation of cellular injury (4).

TABLE 1. Liver NTP contents as measured by NMR or HPLC analyses under various conditions

		37°C Perfusion	4°C Perfusion	4°C Ischémia
NMR	NTP	100%	113±9%	38±10%
HPLC	ATP+GTP+UTP	100%	108±15%	30±6%
	ATP	100%	115%	26%
	GTP	100%	87%	28%
	UTP	100%	74%	65%

Control values (100%) are: NTP, 7.56±0.23 (n=6); ATP+GTP+UTP, 7.92±1.00 (n=7); ATP, 6.31±0.91 (n=7); GTP, 0.79±0.09 (n=7); UTP, 0.82±0.10 (n=7) expressed in μmol/g liver dry weight.

The effect of a period of cold storage (18 to 24 hr) in various preservation media followed by reperfusion, on the liver NMR spectrum was followed. The variations of NTP level and pHi during the experimental protocol are given in figure 2. As expected, cold ischemia induced a progressive decrease of intracellular NTP. Only UW lactobionate and to a lesser extent HTK solutions are able to maintain detectable amount of NTP after 8 hour ischemia (fig 2A). At the end of the ischemic period (24 hr) no NTP were detected in NMR spectra ; a brief reflush with cold oxygenated Krebs medium induced a sharp increase (within 5 min) of NTP. During the reperfusion phase, the transition from 4 to 37°C induced a further recovery of NTP to reach around 90-95% of the initial value, independent of the nature of the preservation medium. Since animal survival was markedly improved with a liver graft preserved for 24 hours in UW compared to EC (10), our results strongly suggest that post ischemic NTP recovery is a necessary but insufficient indicator of liver viability. In addition, the NTP level measured at 8 hour ischemia seems to be a better predictive criterion of liver viability than NTP post ischemic recovery.

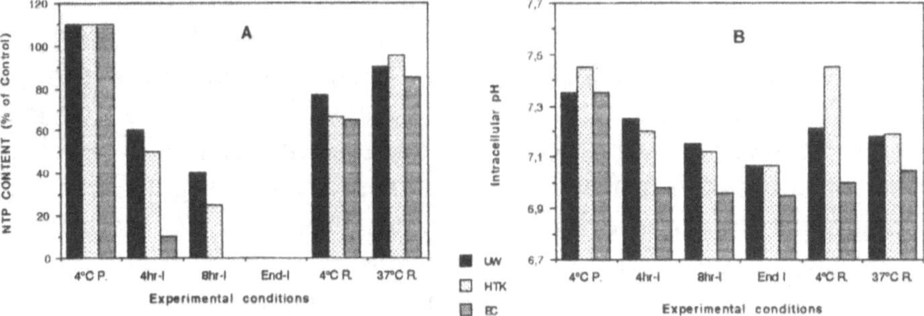

FIG. 2 Variations of intracellular NTP level (A) and intracellular pH (B) in the isolated rat liver during the sequence : perfusion-cold ischemia-reperfusion. NTP levels and pHi are determined from the NMR spectra recorded during the course of the experiment. The liver is perfused for 30 min at 37°C (Control, data not shown) then 15 min at 4°C with Krebs-Henseleit buffer (data not shown) and 15 min at 4°C with the preservation solution (4°C P.).During the cold ischemic storage in preservation solutions, spectra are recorded at 4 hour (4hr-I), 8 hour (8hr-I) and at the end of cold ischemia (End-I). Reperfusion is performed with Krebs medium for 15 min at 4°C, (4°C R.) then the temperature is increased from 4°C to 37°C (37°C R.). Preservation solutions are : Eurocollins (EC), Bretschneider (HTK) and Belzer-lactobionate (UW). The data are given as percent of the initial NTP content.

The intracellular pH of a perfused rat liver is 7.25±0.05 (n=13). For all groups, a higher pHi value was measured at the onset of cold perfusion (figure 2B). During cold ischemia pHi showed a biphasic decay, with a sharp initial fall over the first to second hour of ischemia, followed by a slow decrease over the rest of the cold ischemic period. EC-stored livers showed the lowest pH value at 4 hr (6.98), 8 hr (6.96) and 18 hr (6.85). HTK- and UW-stored livers tended to have the same behaviour with a pHi value in the range of 7.05 at the end of the preservation period. As shown in figure 2B, pHi recovered pre-ischemic values within 5 min of cold reperfusion.

The main results of our work are that (i), the rates of NTP and pHi decrease are strongly dependent on the nature of the preservation solutions, whereas NTP recovery is not significantly different during pos-ischemic reperfusion and (ii), NTP levels after

8 hour-ischemia can be chosen to estimate the performance of the preservation medium. Another important finding is that reperfusion of the preserved liver with a cold synthetic solution can restore pHi and NTP levels almost to control values. This may be of great interest in liver preservation and suggests the possible beneficial effect of successive reflush phases during cold storage. Our results also support the superiority of UW and HTK over EC medium. As previously suggested (11) the combination of histidine and lactobionate solutions has recently proved most effective in animal survival after transplantation (12).

REFERENCES.

1. Desmoulin F., Cozzone P.J. and Canioni P. (1987): *Eur. J. Biochem.,* 162: 151-159.
2. Desmoulin F., Canioni P., Crotte C., Gérolami A. and Cozzone P. (1987): *Hepatology* ,7: 315-323.
3. Delmas-Beauvieux M.C., Gallis J.L., Rousse N., Clerc M. and Canioni P.(1991) *J. of Hepatol.* (in press).
4. Gallis J.L., Delmas-Beauvieux M.C., Biran M., Rousse N., Durand T. and Canioni P. (1991): *NMR in Biomedicine*, (in press).
5. Hutson S.M., Berkich D., Williams G.D., LaNoue K.F. and Briggs R.W. (1989): *Biochemistry,* 28: 4325-4332.
6. Iles R.A., Stevens A.N., Griffiths J.R. and Morris P.G. (1985): *Biochem. J.,* 229: 141-151.
7. Murphy E., Gabel S.A., Funk A., and London R.E. (1988): *Biochemistry* , 27: 526-528.
8. Cohen S.M. (1983): *J. Biol. Chem.*, 23: 14294-14308.
9. Palombo J.D., Hirschberg Y., Pomposelli J.J., Blackburn G.L., Zeisel S.H. and Bistrian B.R. (1988): *Gastroenterology* ,95: 1043-1049
10. Sumimoto R., Jamieson N.V., Wake K. and Kamada N. (1989) : *Transplantation,* 48 : 1-5.
11. Delmas-Beauvieux M.C., Gallis J.L., Clerc M. and Canioni P. (1990) : SMRM, 9th annual meeting, New-York, abstract 2: 953.
12. Sumimoto R., Kamada N., Jamieson N.V., Fukuda Y. and Dohi K.A. (1991): *Transplantation*, 51: 589-593.

DRUGS AND LIVER DISEASE

Sheila Sherlock

Drugs in common use can cause toxic effects on the liver which can mimic almost every naturally occurring liver disease in man (1). About 2% of all cases of jaundice in hospitalized patients are drug-induced. About a quarter of cases of fulminant hepatic failure in the United States are thought to be medicament-related. In any patient with liver disease it is essential to know all drugs that have been taken over the last three months. The physician may have to assume the role of a detective to identify them all. History must include dose, route of administration, duration and any concomitant drugs. Other causes of a hepatic reaction, such as hepatitis A or B or C must be excluded.

Early suspicion of a drug-related hepatic reaction, and, if possible, accurate diagnosis, are essential. Severity is greatly increased if the drug is continued after symptoms develop or after serum aspartate transaminases rise. This provides grounds for negligence claims. The response to a drug depends on absorption and metabolism which are affected by environment and genetics (fig. 1).

HEPATO-CELLULAR ZONE III NECROSIS

Hepato-cellular injury seems to be the primary event, This is rarely due to drug itself and a toxic metabolite is usually responsible (2).

The drug metabolising enzymes activate chemically stable drugs to produce electrophilic metabolites.

These potent alkylating-arylating or acylating agents bind covalently to liver molecules which are essential to the life of the hepatocyte and necrosis ensues. This follows exhaustion of intracellular substances such as glutathione which are capable of preferentially conjugating with a toxic metabolite. In addition, metabolites with an unpaired electron are produced by oxidative reactions of cytochrome P450. These free radicals can also bind covalently to proteins and to the unsaturated fatty acids of cell membranes. This results in lipid perioxidation and membrane damage.

The end-result is hepatocyte deathrelated to failure to pump calcium from the cytosol, and to depressed mitochondrial function.

D. Galmarini et al. (eds.), Drugs and the Liver: High Risk Patients and Transplantation, 91–98.

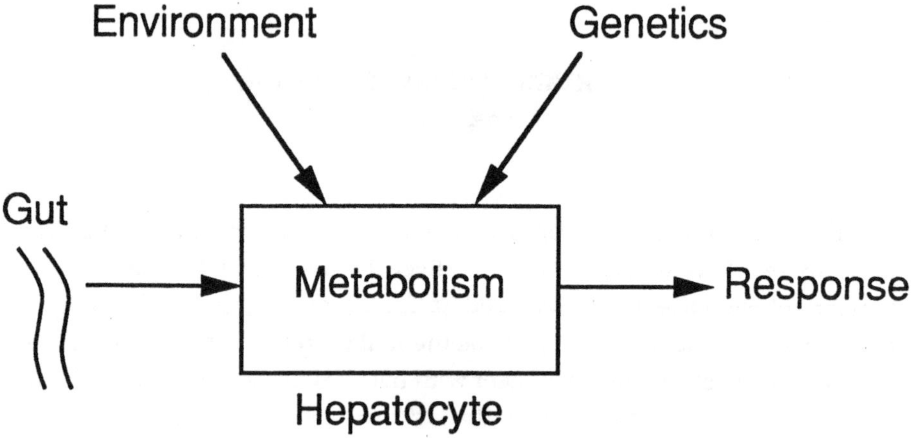

Fig. 1
The response to a drug depends on absorption, metabolism, the environment and genetics

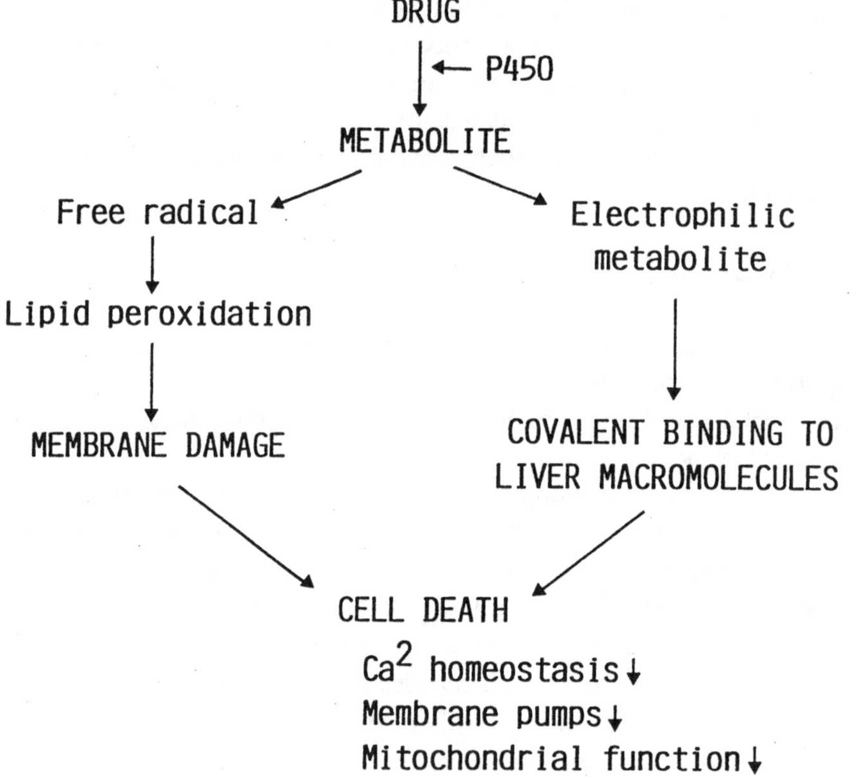

Fig. 2
The mechanism of metabolite-related hepato-toxicity

The P-450 System

Drug metabolism and the production of toxic metabolites is performed by the P-450 system of hemoproteins situated in the endoplasmic reticulum of the hepatocyte. At least 50 P-450's have been identified and there are undoubtedly more. Each P-450 protein is encoded by a unique gene (2).
The human P-450's concerned with drug metabolism are members of three families, P-450 I, P-450 II, and P-450 III. Each P-450 has a unique "substrate" binding site, capable of binding some but not all drugs. Each P-450 can metabolise many drugs.
Genetic differences in the catalytic actitivty of the P-450's may determnine idiosyncratic untoward reactions to drugs. This is exemplified by the poor metabolism of debrisoquine (an anti-arrhythmic drug) due to abnormal expression of P-450-II-D6 (3).
This mechanism also applies to most betablockers and neuroleptics. Poor metabolism of debrisoquine can be identified by PCR amplification of parts of the mutant genes for cytochrome P-450 II D6. This brings up the possibility that in the future those that will react abnormally to a drug can be identified (4). P-450 II E1 is involved in the production of electrophilic metabolites of acetaminophen.

P-450 III A is concerned with the metabolism of cyclosporine and other drugs especially erythromycin, steroids and ketoconazole.
P-450 II C polymorphism affects the metabolism of mephenytoin, diazepam and many other drugs.

Enzyme Induction and Drug Interactions Enzyme induction, by increasing the P-450 enzymes, leads to enhanced production of toxic metabolites.
Expression of P-450's and induction by phenobarbitone are maintained in transplanted hepatocytes without reference to acinar position or zonal sinusoidal microenvironment (5).

Ethanol induces P-450-II E1 and so enhances the toxicity of acetaminophen (fig. 3). Similarly, patients treated with isoniazid which also induces P-450 II E1 have increased acetaminophen toxicity(6).

P-450-III A which metabolites cyclosporin is induced by rifampicin and steroids. This explains the rise in blood cyclosporin levels when these drugs are given. Cyclosporin, erythromycin and ketoconazole compete for binding and metabolism by P-450-III A and cyclosporin levels rise after they are given.

Omeprazole induces P-450 IA (7). This is important in the biotransformation of procarcinogens and carcinogens. An increased tendency to malignancy after omeprazole is possible.

In the future, it should be possible to determine P-450 profiles and detect those likely to develop an adverse drug reaction. Selective inhibitors or inducers may be used to alter the P-450 profile (2).

Immunological Hepatotoxicity The metabolite may act as a hapten with cell protein so inducing immunological liver injury. The P-450's can be involved. Several P-450 isoenzymes are present and inducible on the membranes of hepatocytes and immunization against them might lead to immunological destruction of the liver cell (8).

Halothane metabolites in rats produce antigenically altered members of the P-450-IIB family and this might be the basis of the liver injury following this anaesthetic.

An idiosyncratic reaction to the diuretic, tienilic acid is associated with autoantibodies that react with both liver and kidney microsomes (anti-LKM II). The antigen recognised is within the P-450 IIC family which is also involved in the metabolism of tienilic acid (9).

THE SPECTRUM OF HEPATIC DRUG REACTIONS

Acute Hepato-cellular necrosis is dose dependent and related to a toxic metabolite. Acetaminophen is a good example.

Microvesicular fat syndrome is associated with sodium valproate. It is unusual as it affects children. The toxic metabolite is 4-en-valproate.

Alcoholic Hepatitis This histological picture is associated with amiodarone, a drug with a very long half-life (10). The liver histology is marked by phospholipidosis, a feature also seen with the intra-hepatic cholestasis complicating trimethoprim-sulfamethoxazole therapy (11).

Fibrosis This leads to cirrhosis and is a feature of reactions to cytotoxic drugs especially methotrexate (12). In severe cases, hepatic transplantation may be necessary (13).

Therapeutic vitamin A administration causes a hyperplasia of fat storing (Ito) cells with the appearance of fluorescent vacuoles. Fibrosis and cirrhosis are consequences (14). Retinoid derivatives of vitamin A, including etretinate can also cause hepatic fibrosis and cirrhosis (15).

Acute Hepatitis Picture This resembles virus hepatitis very closely. The reaction usually appears one to six weeks after starting the drug.

It is particularly severe in elderly women. It may be fulminant and treated only by hepatic transplantation. Isoniazid enhanced by rifampicyn induction is a frequent cause (16). The relationship to acetylator status is uncertain. The slow acetylator phenotype is caused by decreased or absent arylamine-N-acetyltransferase (17).

Almost all the non-steroidal, anti-inflammatory drugs have been incriminated. These include piroxicam (18) and particularly diclofenac (19, 20). Others include betablockers such as labetalol (21), tranquillisers, anti-thyroid drugs (22), oral hypoglycaemics (23), sustained-release nicotinic acid (24) and tetrahydroaminoacridine used to treat Alzheimer's disease (25). Etoposide (VP16-213) (26) and cytoproterone (27) are cytotoxic drugs which can cause severe hepatitis.

Hepatic Granulomas Are usually associated with a general hypersensitivity reaction and can complicate therapy with phenylbutazone, carbamazepine and sulphonamides. Allopurinol granulomas may be surrounded by a fibrin ring (28).

Canalicular Cholestasis Is a benign dose-dependent reaction, ususally to steroid sex hormones. It has been reported with cyclosporin which inhibits hepatocyte vesicle transport (29).

It can also complicate treatment with azathioprine and danazol (30).

Hepato-canalicular Cholestasis Is marked by a picture which is cholestatic but has a hepato-cellular component. It is best illustrated by reactions to chlorpromazine, where those affected are poor sulfoxidisers (31). Other members of the group include procarbazine, flucloxacillin (32) and amoxicillin-clavulinate (augmentin) where the reaction is likely to be due to the clavulinic acid (33). Rarely, the bile ductules disappear and the cholestasis becomes chronic. In these circumstances hepatic transplantation mey become necessary.

Biliary Sludge This is a complication of treatment with the antibiotic, ceftriaxone. The sludge consists of small amounts of cholesterol and bilirubin, the major component being the calcium salt of the drug (34). Sludging is related to the sharing with bile acids of a common pathway for hepatic transport and also interactions with biliary lipid excretion (35).

Sclerosing Choangitis Is a consequence of intra-hepatic arterial pump perfusion of cytotoxic agents, particularly FUDR.

Vascular Lesions These complicate treatment usually with cytotoxic drugs or steroid androgens and oestrogens. Veno-occlusive disease is particularly associated with azathioprine and other cytotoxic drugs (36).

Mild sclerosis of some portal zones results in the picture of idiopathic portal hypertension after cytotoxic therapy for leukaemia (37).

Hepatic venous occlusion (Budd-Chiari syndrome) can follow azathioprine immunosuppression after kidney transplantation (38).

Neoplasms These include adenoma, hepato-cellular carcinoma and focal nodular hyperplasia. These are associated particularly with sex hormones, with anabolic steroids and with danazol (39).

Conclusions An iatrogenic cause must be considered in any patient presenting with any clinical pattern of hepato-biliary disease. Some catastrophies would be avoided if clinical trials included subjects of all ages, from children to old people, and those with liver disease. In most instances, challenge is ethically unjustifiable.

However, reporting agencies and drug manufacturers should pay particular attention to the results of inadvertant challenge and to the effects of withdrawing the drug (dechallenge).

REFERENCES

1. Sherlock S. (1986) Lancet, 2; 440-443.
2. Watkins P.B. (1990) Sem. Liver Dis. 10: 235-250.
3. Gonsalez F.J., Skodar R.C., Kimura S. et al. (1988) Nature, 331: 442-446.
4. Heim M., Meyer U.A. (1990) Lancet, 336: 529-532.
5. Magnato P., Traber P.G., Rusnell C. et al. (1990) Hepatology 11: 585-593.
6. Murphy R., Swartz R., Watkins P.B. (1990) Ann. int. Med. 113: 799-800.
7. Diaz D., Fabre I., Daujat M. et al. (1990) Gastroenterology, 99: 737-747.
8. Loper J., Descatoire V., Maurice M. et al. (1989) Hepatology, 10: 610.
9. Beaune P., Dansette P., Mansuy D. et al. (1987) Proc. Natl. Acad. Sci. USA 84: 551-555.
10. Lewis J.H., Ranard R.C., Caruso A. et al. (1989) Hepatology 9: 679-685.
11. Munoz S.J., Martinez-Hernandez A., Maddrey W.C. (1986) Hepatology 12: 342-347.
12. Lewis J.H., Schiff E. (1988) Am. J. Gastroenterol. 12: 1337-1345.
13. Gilbert S.C., Klintmalm G., Silverman A. (1990) Arch. intern. Med. 150: 889-891.
14. Geubel A.P., De Galocsy C., Alves N. et al. (1991) Gastroenterology 100: 1701-1709.

15. Van Ditzhuijsen T.J.M., van Haelst U.J.M., Van Dooren-Greebe R.J. (1990). J. Hepatol. 11: 185-188.
16. Steele M.A., Burk R.F., Des Prez R.M. (1991) Chest 99: 465-471.
17. Grant D.M., Morike K., Eichelbaum M. et al. (1990) J. Clin. Invest. 85: 968-972.
18. Plana S.R., Deleon R., Quer J.C. et al. (1990) Amer. J. Gastroenterol. 85: 468-470.
19. Iveson T.J., Ryley N.G., Kelly P.M.A. et al. (1990) J. Hepatol. 10: 85-89.
20. Helfgott S.M., Sandberg-Cook J., Zakim D. et al. (1990). J. Amer. Med. Ass. 264: 2660-2662.
21. Clark J.A., Zimmerman H.J., Tanner L.A. et al. (1990). Ann.l intern. Med. 113: 210-213.
22. Ozenne G., Manchon N.D., Doucet J. et al. (1989) J. Clin. Gastroenterol. 11: 95-97.
23. Rank J.M., Olson R.C. (1989) Gastroenterology 96: 1607-1608.
24. Mullin G.E., Greenson J.K., Mitchell M.C. (1989) Ann. int. Med. 111: 253-254.
25. Hammel P., Larrey D., Bernuau J. et al. (1990) 12: 329-331.
26. Tran A., Housset C., Boboc B. et al. (1991) J. Hepatol. 12: 36-39.
27. Blake J.C., Sawyerr A.M., Dooley J.S. et al. (1990). Gut 31: 556-557.
28. Stricker B.H.C.K., Blok A.P.R., Babany G. et al. (1989). Gastroenterology 96: 1199-1203.
29. Roman I.D., Monte M.J., Gonzaler-Buitrago J.M. et al. (1990) Hepatology 12: 83-91.
30. Silvo M.O., Reddy K.R., McDonald T. et al. (1989) Am. J. Gastroenterol. 84: 426-428.
31. Watson R.G.P., Olomu A., Clements D. et al. (1988) J. Hepatol. 7: 72-78.
32. Miros M., Walker N., Kerlin P. et al. (1990) Aust. NZ J. Med. 20: 251-253.
33. Reddy K.R., Brillant P., Schiff E.R. (1989) Gastroenterology 96: 1135-1141.
34. Park H.Z., Lees S.P., Schy A.L. (1991) Gastroenterology 100: 1665-1670.
35. Xia Y., Lambert K.J., Schteingart D. et al. (1990) Gastroenterology 99: 454-465.
36. Lemley D.E., De Lacy L.M., Seeff L.B. et al. (1989) Ann. Rheum. Dis. 48: 342-346.
37. Shepherd P., Harrison D.J. (1990) J. Clin. Path. 43: 206-210.

38. Read A.E., Wiesner R.H., La Brecque D.R. (1986) Ann. int. Med. 104: 651-655.

39. Fermand J.P., Levy Y., Bouscary D. et al. (1990) Amer. J. Med. 88: 529-530.

LIVER DISEASE AND ANTICANCER DRUG TREATMENT

G. Powis

INTRODUCTION

Anticancer drugs probably have the smallest therapeutic index of any drugs. They are one of the few classes of therapeutic agents that are routinely given to patients at doses producing moderate to severe toxicity. Significant patient toxicity is closely associated with the use of all the effective anticancer drugs (1). There is good evidence that higher doses of anticancer drugs offer a greater likelihood of therapeutic response and in order to achieve the maximum therapeutic activity significant patient morbidity has to be tolerated (2-4). An unfortunate sequela is that because of human variability there will be some patients who experience severe, even life threatening, toxic responses to the standard doses of anticancer drugs. Clinicians are well used to titrating the dose of anticancer drugs. However, an understanding of the causes of human variability in toxic response to anticancer drugs can go a long way to avoiding unnecessary toxicity and can improve the quality of life of cancer patients. A significant cause of pharmacokinetic variability in the response to anticancer drugs, and one that forms the basis for dose reduction of some anticancer drugs, is liver dysfunction (5).

LIVER DYSFUNCTION IN CANCER PATIENTS

There are several potential causes of liver dysfunction in cancer patients. They are pre-existing liver disease, the cancer drugs themselves, and tumor cell infiltration of the liver. Cancer patients can have many forms of pre-existing liver disease which will not be discussed further here. Cancer drugs themselves can cause liver injury (6,7). For example, hepatocellular necrosis is often seen following the use of L-asparaginase, cytarabine, 6-thioguanine, nitrosoureas, and high doses of methotrexate. Cholestasis can result from treatment with busulfan, anabolic steroids and tamoxifen. Venoocclusive disease is associated with the use of indicine N-oxide, cytarabine, 6-thioguanine, mitomycin C, dacarbazine and daunorubicin. Hydroxyurea treatment can give rise to peliosis hepatitis.

D. Galmarini et al. (eds.), Drugs and the Liver: High Risk Patients and Transplantation, 99–104.

Approximately one-third of patients with malignant disease have metastatic involvement of the liver (8) while approximately half of patients with advanced metastatic disease show an increase in serum liver enzyme levels indicating possible liver dysfunction (9,10). There is some evidence that tumors that metastasize to the liver can lead to a decrease in hepatic drug-metabolizing activity in cancer patients (11-13). It is less clear whether a tumor at a site distant to the liver can lead to altered hepatic drug metabolism in human subjects. Studies in animals have shown that a variety of primary or transplantable solid tumors growing at a site distant to the liver can produce a decrease in the metabolism of a number of drugs including cancer drugs (14,15). However, in these studies large decreases in hepatic drug-metabolizing activity were not seen until the tumor equaled or exceeded 10% of the animal's body weight (16-18). Solid tumors of this size rarely occur in human, and it has been difficult to demonstrate differences in the metabolism of test compounds between cancer patients with solid tumor and carefully matched control subjects (19). Some human hematological tumors such as leukemia and lymphoma can achieve appreciable tumor burdens and infiltrate many tissues, including the liver. We examined whether leukemic cell infiltration of the liver might lead to hepatic dysfunction with decreased drug metabolism using mice injected i.v. with P388 leukemia (20). Changes in liver function were not seen until 8 days after tumor injection when the liver had increased in weight by 50% due to leukemic cell infiltration. At this time there was a 60% decrease in hepatic microsomal cytochrome P-450 and in microsomal mixed function oxygenase activity. There was an increase in serum liver enzymes associated with leukemic cell infiltration of the liver but no change in serum bilirubin. This is similar to the clinical picture of leukemic and lymphoma cell infiltration of the liver in cancer patients (21).The *in vivo* clearance of cyclophosphamide, an anticancer drug metabolized by cytochrome P-450, was decreased by 45% and the metabolism of another anticancer drug, 5-fluorouracil, decreased by 32%. Indocyanine green (ICG) clearance was decreased by 31% suggesting a decrease in hepatic blood flow. A possible explanation for the decrease in drug metabolism is that the hepatocytes were deprived of oxygen and nutrients by the tumor in the liver, coupled with or caused by a physical obstruction of hepatic blood flow.

VINCRISTINE PHARMACOKINETICS NEUROTOXICITY AND LIVER DYSFUNCTION

As a clinical correlate of leukemic cell infiltration of liver in mice described above, we are currently examining the effects of liver dysfunction on vincristine pharmacokinetics and neurotoxicity in lymphoma patients. Vincristine is an alkaloid used extensively in combination with other drugs for the treatment of Hodgkin's and non-Hodgkin's lymphoma (22). Periphenal neuropathy is a frequent and serious toxicity of vincristine which often requires dose reduction or cessation of therapy (23,24). For example, we have found that 17/24 lymphoma patients receiving vincristine experienced some neurotoxicity and 11/24 had severe neurotoxicity. It has been claimed that the incidence of neurotoxicity due to vincristine in patients with lymphoma is much greater than in cancer patients with other malignant diseases (25). Vincristine and its metabolites are excreted primarily in the bile (24,26,27) and neurotoxicity due to vincristine has been reported to be increased in patients with liver dysfunction (28). It has been suggested that the dose of vincristine should be decreased in such patients, but there are no generally accepted guidelines (27). Lymphoma patients frequently have lymphocyte infiltration of the liver and focal hepatic necrosis (29), but without marked alteration in serum chemistry (21). Based on the hypothesis that newer tests of liver function might predict the need for vincristine dose reduction to avoid neurotoxicity, we have initiated an investigation of the possible association between delayed vincristine elimination, neurotoxicity and liver function assessed by serum postprandial total bile acids and the aminopyrine breath test in lymphoma patients. A preliminary summary of results is given in Table 1.

TABLE 1. Liver Function, Vincristine Pharmacokinetics and Neurotoxicity in Lymphoma Patients

Patient	Liver Function[a]			Pharmacokinetics		Neurotoxicity[b] Grade
	Breath Test %/2 hr	Bile Acid μM	Bilirubin mg/dl	t 1/2β hr	Vd l/m2	
1	6.2	11.7	0.8	24.4	428	1
2	4.6	3.1	0.4	17.8	876	0
3	1.0	35.0	2.7	12.4	75	4
4	7.0	3.9	0.4	7.9	66	2
5	6.9	5.4	0.7	4.2	503	2
6	4.9	5.2	0.4	16.8	458	1
7	3.1	2.5	0.5	7.6	368	0

[a] Only subject 3 had biopsy proven liver tumor involvement; [b] 1 = minor; 4 = severe

One patient (#3) in whom liver function measured by serum chemistrywas moderately compromised and who had biopsy proven liver involvement by tumor received a 50% vincristine dose reduction based on elevated bilirubin (per ECOG guidelines). Despite the dose reduction very high plasma concentrations of vincristine due to a decreased apparent volume of distribution (Vd) were observed and the patient developed severe neurotoxicity with paralytic ileus and eventually died of sepsis. Surveying the results shown in Table 1 it is apparent that serum chemistry predicts poorly for neurotoxicity and elevated bilirubin is a particularly poor predictor. The aminopyrine breath test was depressed (< 5%/2 hr) in more than half the patients but predicted poorly for the grade of neurotoxicity. Serum total bile acid was generally elevated (> 5 μM) in patients who experienced more neurotoxicity. Additional patients are being accrued to the study.

DOXORUBICIN DOSE REDUCTION IN LIVER DISEASE

Doxorubicin is a widely used anticancer drug. It is eliminated primarily by the liver as unchanged drug and metabolites (30,31). Benjamin et al. (32) first reported that patients with significantly impaired liver function, measured by

BSP retention, receiving a normal single dose of doxorubicin every 3 weeks, experienced severe and sometimes fatal toxicity with prolonged bone marrow depression and severe mucositis, compared to patients with normal liver function. The increased toxicity was not associated with an increase in the therapeutic efficacy of doxorubicin. Plasma concentrations of doxorubicin and metabolites in the patients with hepatic dysfunction were several fold higher than in patients with normal hepatic function and the elimination of doxorubicin from plasma was delayed (Figure 1). Elimination of doxorubicin metabolites from plasma was also delayed. By reducing the dose of doxorubicin given to patients with hepatic dysfunction, plasma concentrations of doxorubicin and metabolites, response rates and toxicities similar to those in patients with normal liver function receiving full doses of doxorubicin could be obtained. Subsequently, Bachur et al. (33) also showed that it was possible to obtain similar plasma concentrations of doxorubicin and metabolites in patients with normal liver function, and in patients with various degrees of hepatic dysfunction, by decreasing of the dose of doxorubicin given to patients with hepatic dysfunction. Elevated serum bilirubin has been found to be a better predictor of delayed doxorubicin elimination than BSP retention or serum liver enzymes (32,34,35). Benjamin et al. (34) reported three patients with abnormal BSP retention without hyperbilirubinemia, who exhibited normal doxorubicin pharmacokinetics and who could tolerate full doses of doxorubicin. Gisselbrecht et al. (35) found that serum alkaline phosphatase and BSP retention did not predict delayed elimination of doxorubicin. In addition, they reported that serum bilirubin was not always elevated in patients with abnormal doxorubicin kinetics. This has been found by other workers. Doroshow and Chan (36) reported a study of patients with malignant disease involving the liver, where decreased doxorubicin plasma clearance was not predicted by changes in serum bilirubin or serum liver enzymes, although it correlated well with ICG clearance. In this study some patients had clinical evidence of doxorubicin toxicity despite dose reduction according to established guidelines.

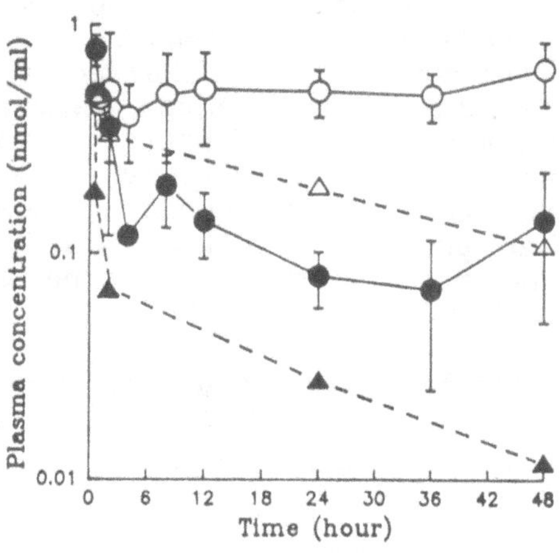

FIG. 1. Plasma doxorubicin and metabolites in cancer patients with normal liver function (triangles and dotted line) and in patients with liver dysfunction (circles and continuous line), (▲, ●) doxorubicin and (△, ○) doxorubicin metabolites. Data redrawn from Benjamin et al. (32).

OTHER ANTICANCER DRUGS SHOWING DECREASED ELIMINATION DUE TO LIVER DYSFUNCTION

There are a number of anticancer drugs whose elimination has been reported to be delayed in patients with liver dysfunction. Some of these drugs are listed in Table 2. It is not general practice to decrease the dose of most of these drugs until toxicity occurs.

TABLE 2. Anticancer Drugs Showing Delayed Elimination in Cancer Patients With Liver Dysfunction

Drug	Pharmacokinetic Parameters[a]	Test of Liver Function[b]
Acivicin	$\uparrow t_{1/2}$, $\downarrow \overline{Cl}$	
Doxorubicin	$\uparrow t_{1/2}$, $\downarrow \overline{Cl}$, $\uparrow C$	B, BSP, E
m-AMSA	$\uparrow t_{1/2}$, $\downarrow \overline{Cl}$	
Cyclophosphamide	$\rightarrow t_{1/2}$	B, E
Dihydroxyanthracenedione	$\uparrow t_{1/2}$, $\downarrow \overline{Cl}$, $\downarrow V_d$	B, E
DTIC	$\uparrow t_{1/2}$	
Etoposide	$\uparrow t_{1/2}$, $\downarrow \overline{Cl}$	B
5-FU	$\uparrow t_{1/2}$, $\rightarrow \overline{Cl}$, $\uparrow C$	E
Ftorafur	$\uparrow t_{1/2}$, $\downarrow \overline{Cl}$, $\uparrow C$, $\rightarrow V_d$	B, E
Melamines	$\uparrow t_{1/2}$	B,E
Melphalan	$\downarrow t_{1/2}$, $\downarrow C$	B
Methotrexate	$\rightarrow t_{1/2}$	B
Mitomycin C	$\uparrow t_{1/2}$	E
PALA	$\uparrow t_{1/2}$, $\uparrow \overline{Cl}$, $\downarrow C$, $\uparrow V_d$	B, E
Vincristine	$\uparrow t_{1/2}$, $\downarrow \overline{Cl}$, $\rightarrow V_d$	A

[a]$t_{1/2}$, post-distributive half-life; $\overline{Cl}$ total body plasma clearance; V_d, apparent volume of distribution; C, plasma concentration
[b]A, elevated serum alkaline phosphatase; BSP, increased bromosulphthalein retention; E, increased serum liver enzymes

REFERENCES

1. Powis G. (1991): The Toxicity of Anticancer Drugs. Pergamon Press, New York.
2. DeVita V.T. (1989): In: Cancer Principles and Practice of Oncology, edited by V.T. DeVita, S. Hellman, and S.A. Rosenberg pp. 276-300. Lippincott, Philadelphia.
3. Frei E., Canellas G.P. (1980): Am. J. Med., 69: 585-594.
4. Gehan E.A. (1984): Cancer, 54: 1204-1207.

5. Powis G. (1983): Pharmacokinetics of anticancer agents in humans. Elsevier, Amsterdam.
6. McDonald G.B., Tirumali N. (1984): West. J. Med., 140: 250-259.
7. Zimmerman H.J. (1988): Prog. Liver Dis., 8: 621-642.
8. Ozarda A., Pickren J. (1962): J. Nucl. Med., 3: 149-152.
9. Mendelsohn M.L., Bodansky O. (1952): Cancer, 5: 1-7.
10. Schaefer J., Schiff L. (1965): Gastroenterology, 49: 360-363.
11. Hepner G.W., Uhlin S.R., Lipton A., Harvey H.A., Rohrer G.V. (1976): J. Am. Med. Assoc., 236: 1587-1590.
12. Higuchi Z., Nakamura T., Uchino H. (1980): Cancer, 45: 541-544.
13. Pelkonen O., Karki N.T., Larmi T.K.I. (1973): Chir. Gastroenterol., 7: 436-443.
14. Kato R. (1963): Experientia, 19: 31-32.
15. Bartosek I., Donelli M.G., Guaitani A., Colombo T., Russo R., Garattini S. (1975): Biochem. Pharmacol., 24: 289-291.
16. Kato R., Takanaka A., Takahashi H., Onoda K. (1968): Jpn. J. Pharmacol., 18: 224-244.
17. Rosso R., Dolfini E., Donelli M.G. (1968): Eur. J. Cancer, 4: 133-135.
18. Rosso R., Donelli M.G., Franchi G., Garattini S. (1971): Eur. J. Cancer, 7: 565-577.
19. Tschanz C., Hignite C.E., Huffman D.A., Azarnoff D.L. (1977): Cancer Res., 37: 3881-3886.
20. Powis G., Harris R.N., Basseches P.J., Santone K.S. (1986): Cancer Chemother. Pharmacol., 16: 43-49.
21. Friedman R.B., Anderson R.E., Entine S.M., Hirshberg S.B. (1980): Clin. Chem., 26(Suppl.): 1-475.
22. Dorr R.T., Fritz W.L. (1980): In: Handbook of Cancer Chemotherapy, pp. 685-691. Elsevier, New York.
23. Holland J.F., Scharlau C., Gailani S., Krant M.J., Olson K.B., Horton J., Shnider B.I., Lynch J.J., Owens A., Carbone P.P., Grob D., Miller S.P., Hall T.C. (1973): Cancer Res., 33: 1258-1264.
24. Sandler S.G., Tobin W., Henderson E.S. (1969): Neurology, 19: 367-374.
25. Watkins S.M., Griffin J.P. (1978): Br. Med. J., 1: 610-612.
26. Jackson D.V., Castle M.C., Bender R.A. (1978): Clin. Pharmacol. Ther., 24: 101-107.
27. Bender R.A., Zwelling L.A., Doroshow J.H., Locker G.Y., Hande K.R., Murinson D.S., Cohen M., Myers C.E., Chabner B.A. (1978): Drugs, 16: 46-87.
28. Mueller J.M., Flaherty M.J. (1978): South. Med. J., 71: 1301-1311.
29. Edmonson J.A., Peters R.L. (1982): In: Diseases of the Liver, edited by L. Schiff and E.R. Schiff pp. 1101-1140.
30. Glode L.M., Israel M., Pegg W.J., Wilkinson P.M. (1977): Br. J. Clin. Pharmacol., 4: 639.
31. Riggs C.E., Benjamin R.S., Serpick A.A., Bachur N.R. (1977): Clin. Pharmacol. Ther., 22: 234-241.
32. Benjamin R.S., Wiernik P.H., Bachur N.R. (1974): Cancer, 33: 19-27.
33. Bachur N.R., Riggs C.E., Green M.R., Langore M.R., Van Vurakis J.J., Levine L. (1977): Clin. Pharmacol. Ther., 21: 70-77.
34. Benjamin R.S., Loo T.L., Friedman J., Ho D.H., Rodriquez V., Gottlieb J.A., Freireich E.J. (1975): Pharmacologist, 17: 265.
35. Gisselbrecht C., Likiec F., Marty M., Mignot L., Belpomme D., Najean Y., Boiron M. (1980): Cancer Chemother. Pharmacol., 5(Suppl.): 20.
36. Doroshow J., Chan K. (1982): Proc. Am. Assoc. Clin. Oncol., 1: 11.

PHARMACOKINETICS OF ANTICANCER AGENTS IN PATIENTS WITH IMPAIRED LIVER FUNCTION

Maria Grazia Donelli, Massimo Zucchetti, Donatella Gentili and Maurizio D'Incalci.

The narrow therapeutic index and the potentially life-threatening toxicities of anticancer agents makes a proper pharmacokinetic information on the time course of a drug and its metabolites in the body crucial in the development of rational dosage regimens. As a pathological situation may affect drug disposition and cancer patients usually suffer from a series of diseases unrelated to the neoplastic process, it is important to have information on the clinical pharmacokinetics of antitumoral agents in the presence of one or more specific pathologies.

Liver disease has a profound and unpredictable effect on drug kinetics by altering the intrinsic hepatic clearance, by reducing the metabolic capacity or affecting excretion in the bile, by reducing serum protein binding or affecting absorption from the gastrointestinal tract. In cancer patients the etiology of hepatic failure (HF) may be due to other diseases affecting the liver such as hepatitis or cirrhosis, to toxicity induced by chemotherapy or to deterioration of general liver function in the presence of a neoplastic process inside or outside the liver tissue. Impairment of drug clearance can be related to stasis of the hepatic blood flow induced by the presence of liver metastases compressing the hepatocyte or to an intrinsic reduced metabolizing capacity of the hepatocyte not always resulting in clearly modified parameters of the liver function.

D. Galmarini et al. (eds.), Drugs and the Liver: High Risk Patients and Transplantation, 105–111.

The role of the liver and of altered hepatic function is particularly significant for anticancer drugs which undergoe hepatobiliary elimination or extensive biotransformation, either producing active metabolites (e.g. cyclophosphamide, dacarbazine) or resulting in detoxified products (e.g. doxorubicin, mitoxantrone, vinca alkaloids). For drugs which are highly protein-bound (e.g. etoposide or anthracycline antibiotics) a condition of hypoalbuminaemia, frequently arising in liver disease, increases the fraction of unbound drug responsible for drug effects.

Increased toxicity associated or not to delayed drug clearance in cancer patients showing some altered biochemical tests of liver function has been described for a series of anticancer agents (1). To avoid toxicity drastic dose reductions have been often suggested, without considering the steep dose-response curve for these drugs and the consequent danger of underdosing. However reliable dosage modifications schemes, based on detailed pharmacology studies of plasma concentration for a given patient in the presence of HF, are mostly not described or lack consistent evidence.

We will briefly review the literature on the pharmacokinetics of four widely used antitumor agents, doxorubicin, cyclophosphamide, etoposide and vincristine in cancer patients with HF, chosen as examples of drugs for which the question of dosage adjustment in the presence of altered liver function tests has frequently arisen.

For doxorubicin (DX) the conventional guideline for the clinical practice is based on early reports (2) describing delayed drug elimination in the presence of HF. The dose of DX should be reduced by 50% if serum bilirubin ranges between 2 and 3 mg/100ml and treatment should be withheld in patients with bilirubin > 5mg/100ml.

However subsequent studies by other authors, Chan et al (3), Chlebowski et al (4), Peterson et al (5), Preiss et al (6) failed to confirm these results. In patients with hepatoma and proven cirrhosis or with liver metastases, showing abnormal bilirubin and serum liver enzymes, the profiles of DX levels were always apparently normal but delayed appearance and prolonged half-life of doxorubicinol was observed in all studies. Moreover in patients undergoing conventional dose reduction suggested for HF, duration of response and survival result decreased in spite of a lower drug-induced toxicity. The finding by Preiss (6) that the elimination rate of DX correlate with the corresponding parameter for antipyrine, used as marker for the liver monooxygenase metabolizing capacity, but not with usual liver function tests is of difficult interpretation, due to the different elimination mechanisms of the two drugs. On the basis of these studies it would thus appear that in patients with HF only a small dose adjustment should be done to avoid underdosing.

The pharmacokinetics of cyclophosphamide (CTX) in patients with HF has been investigated in previous reports by Bagley et al (7). The results of subsequent studies by Wagner et al (8) and by Juma (9) in patients showing altered bilirubin, albumin and serum liver enzymes due to metastatic deposits in the liver are summarized in Table 1.

TABLE 1 PHARMACOKINETICS OF CYCLOPHOSPHAMIDE IN CANCER PATIENTS WITH HEPATIC FAILURE.

Study	Drug and Dose mg/sq.m or kg i.v.	Patients nr. with HF/total	Test of Liver function	Pharmacokinetic behaviour
Von Wagner (1980)	2.5-20/kg	Ca. with met. (10)	CHE	Cls (ml/min) 118±34 in C 67±20 in H.F. β t1/2 (h) 4.3±0.7 in C 6.7±1.1 in H.F. AUC of activated metabolites (nmol/ml x h) 9.9±3.5 in C 8.6±3.9 in H.F.
Juma (1984)	15/kg	Hodgkin disease (7/17)	BIL SGOT ALB	Cls (l/kg) 63±7.6 in C 44.8±5.6 in H.F. β t1/2 (h) 7.6±1.4 in C 12.5±1 in H.F.

BIL= bilirubin
ALB= albumin
SGOT= transaminase
A PH= alkaline phosphatase
CHE= colinesterase
γGT=γ glutaminil transferase
ca.= carcinoma
met.= metastases
pts.= patients
C.= controls with normal liver function

This compound, which undergoes extensive biotransformation to the active metabolite 4-OHCTX and then to the inactive 4-ketoCTX and 4-carbossiCTX in the liver (10), should be sensitive to changes in the hepatic function. However in patients with HF reduced clearance and prolonged half-life of CTX as well as delayed appearance of 4-OHCTX, being the total clearance of CTX function of hepatic metabolism and not of urinary elimination, do not result in changes in the overall exposure to the active metabolites. In agreement with this pharmacokinetic finding no clinical evidence of increased toxicity was observed by Juma (9) in patients with liver dysfunction and thus apparently no dosage adjustment is recommended in the presence of HF.

Another widely used antitumor compound, whose pharmacokinetics in the presence of organ failure has been the object of investigation, is the epipodophyllotoxin etoposide (VP16). Clearance of VP16 in humans occurs both by direct excretion or metabolism to the inactive glucuronide derivatives (11, 12). It has been speculated that impairment of the hepatic function may decrease the rate of VP16 metabolism and/or biliary excretion, thus increasing toxicity. Although no pharmacokinetic and toxicity data are available to support this speculation, dose reduction of VP16 is often usual clinical practice in patients with elevated bilirubin.

TABLE 2 PHARMACOKINETICS OF ETOPOSIDE IN CANCER PATIENTS WITH HEPATIC FAILURE.

Study	Drug and Dose mg/sq.m or kg i.v.	Patients nr. with HF/total	Test of Liver function	Pharmacokinetic behaviour
Arbuck (1986)	100x3	Hepatobiliary tumor (8/17)	BIL	Cls (ml/min/sq.m.) 21.4±7.4 in C 22.4±9.6 in H.F. β t1/2 (h) 8.1±2.8 in C 8.4±3.9 in H.F.
D'Incalci (1986)	80-150 x 1 or 3	Hepatoca. or extrahepatic tumors with/without liver met. (15/33)	BIL γGT A PH	Cls (ml/min/sq.m.) 22.8±1.0 in C 27.9±2.7 in H.F. β t1/2 (h) 5.6±0.4 in C 5.4±0.6 in H.F.
Hande (1990)	100-800	Obstructive jaundice in pts. with cancer (10/33)	BIL SGOT A PH	Cls (ml/min/sq.m.) 26.5±9.8 in C 24.5±6.5 in H.F. β t1/2 (h) 6.4±2.5 in C 5.7±1.5 in H.F.

See legend under Table 1

Table 2 describes the results of three studies on the pharmacokinetics of VP16 in the presence or absence of HF, which are strikingly superimposable. Arbruck et al (13), D'Incalci et al (14) of our group and Hande et al (15) were not able to evidentiate differences in the clearance and half-life of VP16 between patients with normal liver function and patients with altered bilirubin or liver enzymes due to primary or secondary liver neoplasms with or without obstructive jaundice. Metaanalysis of the combined data (mean clearance being 24.3 vs. 25.3 ml/min/sq.m and half-life 6.4 vs. 6.3 hours in patients with normal vs. impaired liver function respectively) clearly indicate that the pharmacokinetics of VP16 is not significantly altered in the presence of HF (15). On the basis of the information outlined in these pharmacokinetic studies normal doses of VP16 should be given to patients with HF. In this regard it is worthy of mention that increased pharmacologic effects of standard VP16 doses could be theoretically determined by changes in protein binding of etoposide and higher levels of unbound (active) drug at any given total drug concentration observable in cancer patients as compared to normal volunteers (16).

Finally we will briefly discuss about Vincristine (VCR), which seems a clear example of antitumor agent requiring dose adjustment in cancer patients with impaired liver function.

A consistent finding in clinical trials after repeated administrations of VCR is development of neurotoxicity, which is related to its cumulative dose. As the biliary system represents the principal route or excretion of VCR and its desacethyl-metabolic products (17), it is reasonable to expect that hepatic dysfunction might alter elimination kinetics and increase exposure to the drug and its metabolites, thus increasing toxicity. In spite of significant interindividual variations in the pharmacokinetics of VCR, the plasma clearance in humans has been shown to increase as a function of the dose (18).

TABLE 3 PHARMACOKINETICS OF VINCRISTINE IN CANCER PATIENTS WITH HEPATIC FAILURE.

Study	Drug and Dose mg/sq.m or kg i.v.	Patients nr. with HF/total	Test of Liver function	Pharmacokinetic behaviour
Van Der Berg (1982)	0.4-1.5/sq.m.	Different tumors (15/39)	A PH BIL (3pts)	β t1/2 (h) 5.1±3.5 in C 13.0±10.1 in H.F. AUC (ng/ml/h) 54±3.5 in C 145±88 in H.F.
Desai (1982)	1.4-2/sq.m.	Leukemia and lymphoma (5/16)	A PH	AUC (ng/ml/h) 65±39 in C 197.4±84.5 in H.F. Correlation between dose, AUC and neuropathy.

See legend under Table 1

Table 3 illustrates the results of an Irish group, Van der Berg et al (19) and Desai et al (20), who investigated the pharmacokinetic behaviour of VCR in patients with different tumors showing altered bilirubin and alkaline phosphatase level. As compared to patients with normal liver function, in patients with HF given the same standard doses of the compound, the half-life of VCR is more than doubled and the total availability, as expressed by the area under the concentration versus time curve, results three times higher. Neurotoxicity was found to correlate with dose and plasma AUC and susceptibility to the toxic effects of VCR differ accordingly from patient to patient. It was also observed that in patients with HF a small reduction in the drug dose results in lower VCR plasma AUC and less neurotoxicity (20).

It is therefore reasonable to recommend dose adjustment guided by clinical evidence of toxicity, particularly in view of the observation that dicontinuation of therapy (21) reverses development of neurotoxicity.

In conclusion, with the exception of VCR, the information available in the literature on the pharmacokinetics of most clinically used antineoplastic agents indicates that the clearance of these compounds does not appear to be substantially modified in presence of altered hepatic function and does not necessarily account for dose adjustment. We think that, although caution in treating patients with impaired organ function is compulsory, consideration of the risks of excessive toxicities should not compromise the opportunity for a therapeutic benefit.

REFERENCES

1. Powis G. (1982): Cancer Treat. Rev., 9: 85-124.
2. Benjamin R.S. (1974): Cancer Chemother. Rep., 58: 271-273.
3. Chan K.K., Chlebowski R.T., Tong M., Chen H-S. G., Gross J.F., Bateman J.R. (1980): Cancer Res., 40: 1263-1268.
4. Chlebowski R.T., Chan K.K., Tong M.J., Weiner J.M., Ryden V.M.J., Bateman J.R. (1981): Cancer, 48: 1088-1095.
5. Peterson C., Gunvén P., Theve N-O. (1986): Cancer Treat. Rep., 70: 947-952.
6. Preiss R., Matthias M., Shor R., Brockmann B., Huller H. (1987): J. Cancer Res. Clin Oncol., 113: 593-598.
7. Bagley C.M., Bostick F.W., De Vita V.D. (1973): Cancer Res. 33: 226-235.
8. Wagner V.T., Heydrich D., Bartels H., Hohorst H.J. (1980): Arzneim.-Forsch./Drug Res., 30: 1588-1592.
9. Juma F.D. (1984): Eur. J. Clin. Pharmacol., 26: 591-593.
10. Fenselau C., Kan M-N.N., Rao S.S., Myles A., Friedman O.M., Colvin M. (1977): Cancer Res., 37: 2538-2543.
11. Hande K., Anthony L., Hamilton R., Bennett R., Swéetman B., Branch R. (1988): Cancer Res., 48: 1829-1834.
12. Colombo T., D'Incalci M., Donelli M.G., Bartosek I., Benfenati E., Farina P., Guaitani A. (1985): Xenobiotica, 15: 343-350.
13. Arbuck S.G., Douglass H.O., Crom W.R., Goodwin P., Silk Y., Cooper C. Evans W.E. (1986): J. Clin. Oncol., 4: 1690-1695.
14. D'Incalci M., Rossi C., Zucchetti M., Urso R., Cavalli F., Mangioni C., Willems Y., Sessa C. (1986): Cancer Res., 46: 2566-2571.
15. Hande K.R., Wolff S.N., Greco A., Hainsworth J.D., Reed G., Johnson D.H. (1990): J. Clin. Oncol., 8: 1101-1108.
16. Stewart C.F., Pieper J.A., Arbuck S.G., Evans W.E. (1989): Clin. Pharmacol. Ther., 45: 49-55.

17. Jackson D.V., Castle M.C., Bender R.A. (1978): Clin. Pharmacol. Ther., 24: 101-107.
18. Sethi V.S., Jackson D.V., White D.R., Richards II F., Stuart J.J., Muss H.B., Cooper M.R., Spurr C.L. (1981): Cancer Res., 41: 3551-3555.
19. Van den Berg H.W., Desai Z.R., Wilson R., Kennedy G., Bridges J.M., Shanks R.G. (1982): Cancer Chemother. Pharmacol., 8: 215-219.
20. Desai Z.R., Van den Berg H.W., Bridges J.M., Shanks R.G. (1982): Cancer Chemother. Pharmacol., 8: 211-214.
21. Rosenthal S., Kaufman S. (1974): Ann. Intern. Med., 80: 733-737.

PATHOGENESIS AND TREATMENT OF ALCOHOLIC LIVER DISEASE

Charles S. Lieber, M.D.

The strategy for the treatment of alcoholic liver disease first involved identification of the etiologic agent. Up to 1960, the concept prevailed that the liver disease was due not to the toxicity of alcohol but rather to the dietary deficiencies commonly associated with alcoholism. Since then, epidemiologic, clinical and experimental studies have clearly established the role of the hepatotoxicity of alcohol. Next, major efforts have been directed at defining and controlling the damage produced.

Evidence for the Etiologic Role of Ethanol in the Pathogenesis of Alcoholic Liver Injury

The original view that ethyl alcohol was not more toxic to the liver than sugar was based largely on experimental work in rats given ethanol in drinking water (1). With this technique, however, ethanol consumption does not usually exceed 10-20% of the total caloric intake of the animal. A comparable or even greater amount of alcohol, when given with an adequate diet, resulted in negligible ethanol levels in the blood (2,3). By incorporating ethanol in a totally liquid diet, the amount of ethanol consumed was increased to 36% of total energy; isocaloric replacement of carbohydrate or fat by ethanol in these nutritionally adequate diets consistently produced a 5- to 10-fold increase in hepatic triglycerides (2,3), with associated ultrastructural changes in mitochondria and endoplasmic reticulum (4) and plasma membranes (5), whereas no such lesions developed in pair-fed control animals. The ultrastructural lesions of the mitochondria has a functional counterparts in terms of striking impairment of respiration and energy production (6,7), fatty acid oxidation (8) and susceptibility to acetaldehyde toxicity (9). Continuous intragastric infusion of alcohol-containing liquid diets to rats also resulted in some fibrosis whereas animals given isocaloric amounts of the control diet remained normal (10). However, regarding alcohol-induced fibrosis in the liver, the baboon mimicks the human lesion more closely than the rodent. In the aggregate of all our studies conduced thus fat (11-14), production of cirrhosis was observed in 13 of a total of 63 baboons fed ethanol for 5 years or more, with septal fibrosis developing in an additional 13 animals. No lesions developed in the corresponding pair-fed controls.

The hepatotoxicity for alcohol has also been demonstrated in man. In a series of controlled studies conducted under metabolic ward conditions, it was shown that individuals with a morphologically normal liver developed a fatty liver when given ethanol either in addition to a normal diet, or as an isocaloric substitution for carbohydrates in a variety of non-deficient diets (2,3). This was evident both by morphologic examination (2,3) and by direct measurement of the lipid content of the liver biopsies (15-17). Even with a high protein, vitamin-supplemented diet, there were significant increases in hepatic triglycerides (15). Electron microscopic studies conducted in many of the above cited investigations, as well as by Lane and Lieber (18), showed that alcohol also caused a striking organelle injury, especially to the mitochondria and the endoplasmic reticulum.

D. Galmarini et al. (eds.), Drugs and the Liver: High Risk Patients and Transplantation, 113–118.

The etiologic role of alcohol was also demonstrated in epidemiologic studies. As reviewed elsewhere (19), a variety of studies have clearly linked the incidence of cirrhosis and associated mortality to the amount and duration of alcohol consumed. Of course, factors other than ethanol play a role, such as genetic make-up, viruses, other toxins and dietary composition. In particular, the influence of other hepatotoxins (20) and malnutrition (21) in alcoholic liver disease has been well recognized. However, in addition to these other factors, and even in their absence, ethanol and/or its metabolite acetaldehyde exert hepatotoxic effects, part of which have now been defined.

Pathogenesis of Alcohol-induced Liver Damage

One of the most fruitful approaches to alcoholic liver injury resulted from the unraveling of the link of the various hepatic and metabolic complications of alcoholism to the metabolism of ethanol. This compound, unlike other drugs, is consumed in massive amounts that readily overwhelm the liver's capacity for detoxification. The primary pathway for ethanol metabolism involves hepatic cytosolic alcohol dehydrogenase (ADH) isozymes (22). Extrahepatic tissues also contain isozymes of ADH, but these have a much lower affinity for ethanol than the hepatic ones; as a consequence, at the levels of ethanol achieved in the blood; these extrahepatic enzymes are inactive and therefore, extrahepatic metabolism of ethanol is negligible, with the exception of the gastric one. At least three different forms of ADH exist in the stomach, with either high or low K_m's for ethanol (23). Because of the extraordinary high gastric ethanol concentration after alcohol ingestion, even the gastric ADH with the high K_m for ethanol becomes active and significant gastric ethanol metabolism ensues (24,25). This decreases the bioavailability of ethanol and represents a "protective barrier" against its systemic effects. This barrier disappears after gastrectomy (26) and may be lost, in part, in the alcoholic (27), because of a decrease in gastric ADH. Similar effects may also result from gastric ADH inhibition by some commonly used drugs. For instance aspirin (28), or H_2-blockers, such as cimetidine (29) and ranitidine (30), were found to inhibit gastric ADH activity and to result in increased blood levels when alcohol was consumed in amounts equivalent to social drinking. Under these conditions, famotidine, an equally effective H_2-blocker, did not have this adverse effect (23). Women also have a lower gastric ADH activity than men: as a consequence, for a given intake, their blood ethanol levels are higher (31), an increase that is compounded by differences in body composition (more fat, less water in women) and, on the average, a lower body weight.

In ADH-mediated oxidation of ethanol, acetaldehyde is produced and hydrogen is transferred from ethanol to the cofactor nicotinamide adenine dinucleotide (NAD), which is converted to its reduced form (NADH) (22). The acetaldehyde produced again loses hydrogen and is converted to acetate, most of which is released into the bloodstream. The large amounts of reducing equivalents produced overwhelm the hepatocyte's ability to maintain redox homeostasis and a number of metabolic disorders ensue. These include alterations in the metabolism of lipids, carbohydrates, proteins, and purines (22).

Ethanol is also oxidized in liver microsomes by an ethanol-inducible cytochrome P-450 (32-34), that contributes to ethanol metabolism and tolerance, and activates xenobiotics to toxic radicals, thereby explaining the increased vulnerability of the heavy drinker to industrial solvents, anesthetic agents, commonly prescribed drugs, over-the-counter analgesics, chemical carcinogens, and even nutritional factors, such as vitamin A (22). The specific form of cytochrome P450, involved (P450IIE1), has now been purified, both in rabbits (35) and in man (36).

All known pathways of ethanol oxidation in the liver result in production of acetaldehyde, which in turn is metabolized to acetate. Other hepatotoxic agents have been shown to act through an active metabolite that either promotes lipid peroxidation or covalently binds to proteins. Acetaldehyde, the active metabolite of ethanol, may do both (22), with alterations in microtubules, plasma membranes and mitochondria, and the formation of protein adducts, resulting in antibody production, enzyme inactivation, and decreased DNA repair. Binding of acetaldehyde with cysteine and/or glutathione, inhibition of GSH synthesis and loss from the liver, all contribute to a depression of liver glutathione (37). Ethanol-induced depletion of glutathione has been shown to be particularly striking in primates (37,38). Glutathione offers one of the mechanisms for the scavenging of toxic free radicals. Although GSH depletion is not necessarily sufficient to cause lipid peroxidation, it is generally agreed upon that it may favor the peroxidation produced by other factors. As for tissue damage due to other etiologic agents, alcohol-induced liver damage causes a fibrotic response which, when excessive may result in scarring culminating in cirrhosis. The scarring process can also be promoted by the inflammatory cell reaction which is associated with liver injury, and may also be directly influenced by acetaldehyde itself. Indeed, acetaldehyde was found to increase collagen production in cultured myofibroblasts (39) and Ito cells or fat-storing cells (40), in association with an increase in mRNA of collagen (41).

Repair of Alcohol-induced Liver Damage

Duce et al. (42) reported a decrease in S-adenosyl-L-methionine (SAMe) synthetase and phospholipid methyltransferase activities in cirrhotic livers. Furthermore, long term alcohol consumption was found to be associated with enhanced methionine utilization and depletion (43), as well as depletion of hepatic SAMe (38). Potentially, a significant reduction of SAMe may have a number of adverse effects. SAMe is the principal methylating agent in various vital transmethylation reactions which have been known for some time to be important to nucleic acid and protein synthesis and cell membrane function. Thus, depletion of SAMe, by being detrimental to methyltransferase activity, may promote the membrane injury which has been documented in alcohol-induced liver damage (5). SAMe also plays a key role in the synthesis of polyamines and provides a source of cysteine for glutathione production. Experimentally, the GSH depletion could be corrected, in part, by the administration of SAMe (38). Moreover, SAMe plays an essential role in phospholipid metabolism and the maintenance of membrane structure and function (44).

Excess methionine was shown to have some adverse effects (45) including a decrease in hepatic ATP (46). Compared to methionine, administration of SAMe has the advantage of bypassing the deficit in SAMe synthesis from methionine referred to above. This deficit is due to a decrease in enzyme activity, not in the substrate, and therefore cannot simply be corrected by excess methionine. Replenishment of the hepatocyte with SAMe is feasible through ingestion of the compound; it has been shown that blood concentrations of SAMe are increased after oral administration in rodents (47) and in man (48). Although it has been claimed that the liver does not take up SAMe from the bloodstream (49), other results have indicated uptake of SAMe by isolated hepatocytes either at pharmacological (50) or physiological (51,52) extracellular concentrations. The hepatic SAMe transport system appears to be saturable (52,53). Recent results in baboons (38) also clearly indicate hepatic uptake of exogenous SAMe. Orally administered SAMe may play a precursor role for intracellular SAMe both as unchanged SAMe and also by the methionine it provides. Since the SAMe transport system does not appear to be saturated under physiological conditions, it is likely that SAMe levels in biological compartments regulate, at least in part, the rate of transport across membranes. Indeed, hepatic levels of SAMe are increased with increasing extracellular levels (51) and the intracellular concentrations reached are above or close to the K_m for SAMe of both phospholipid methyltransferase (54) and catechol-*O*-methyltransferase (55). Furthermore, the effective utilization of SAMe both for transmethylation and transulphuration has been demonstrated *in vivo* (56). In the baboon model (38),

SAMe attenuates ethanol-induced liver injury, as shown by lesser increases in plasma aspartate transaminase and glutamic dehydrogenase activities, and fewer ethanol-induced megamitochondria. Thus, alcoholic liver injury may now be added to those other forms of liver disease favorably influenced by SAMe treatment (38,57).

Attenuation of the Excessive Inflammatory and Fibrotic Responses

As for many other disease states, adrenocorticosteroids have been used to limit the inflammatory response caused by alcoholic liver injury. However, the role of adrenocorticosteroid therapy in acute alcoholic hepatitis has been the subject of debate for many years, and is not as yet settled. The most dramatic liver consequence of excess alcohol consumption is the development of excess scar tissue, resulting ultimately in cirrhosis with obstruction to blood flow, portal hypertension, and disastrous clinical consequences. Fibrous tissue is characterized by excess collagen. Collagen accumulation reflects an imbalance between collagen degradation and collagen production. In baboons given ethanol that developed significant fibrosis, molecular evaluation revealed that type I procollagen mRNA content was significantly increased. Cirrhosis might, in part, represent a relative failure of collagen degradation to keep pace with synthesis. The mechanisms of collagen degradation in the liver are complex. During the early stage of alcoholic liver injury collagenolytic activity may be increased (58), together with enhanced collagen synthesis (59). Subsequently, collagenase activity may decrease and contribute to the collagen accumulation (60). Interestingly, addition of polyunsaturated lecithin (PUL) to transformed lipocytes was found to prevent the acetaldehyde-mediated increase in collagen accumulation, possibly by stimulation of collagenase activity (61). If we can extrapolate from these *in vitro* data to the *in vivo* condition, these findings could explain, at least in part, why PUL attenuates the accumulation of collagen after chronic alcohol administration (13), and why, upon withdrawal of PUL, collagen synthesis, still turned on by the ethanol-derived acetaldehyde, but not sufficiently opposed by the resting collagenase, then results in accelerated collagen deposition (13). PUL contains choline, the lack of which has been incriminated before in alcohol-induced liver damage. Choline, however, is responsible for the PUL effect since amounts of choline identical with those provided by PUL had no protective action (12).

Short term treatment of alcoholic liver disease with propylthiouracil has yielded conflicting results, but a more recent long term study reported a reduced mortality (62). Curiously, the beneficial effect was not observed in patients with high alcohol consumption; it was restricted to those in whom alcohol intake was moderate, a group known to have a good outcome even without specific treatment. The mechanism of the beneficial effect is not clear. Propylthiouracil has been shown, experimentally, to protect against alcohol-induced hepatocellular necrosis in hypoxic conditions but such conditions were not documented in the patients who reportedly benefitted, and experimentally, defective oxygen utilization, rather than a lack of blood oxygen supply, characterizes ethanol-induced chronic liver injury (63). Colchicine, which inhibits collagen synthesis and procollagen secretion in embryonic tissue, may provide an alternative for the treatment of alcoholic liver injury (64), and is being further investigated.

In conclusion, the recently gained understanding of the pathophysiology of alcohol-induced liver damage now suggests new avenues for therapeutic interventions. In particular, S-adenosyl-L-methionine (SAMe) and polyunsaturated lecithin may provide long awaited tools to abate some of the hepatotoxic effects of alcohol, and/or the excessive response of the liver to the injury.

References

1. Best C.H., Hartroft W.S., Lucas C.C. and Ridout J.H. (1949): *Br. Med. J.* 2: 1001-1006.

2. Lieber C.S., Jones D.P., Mendelson J. and DeCarli L.M. (1963): *Trans. Assoc. Am. Physicians* 76: 289-300.
3. Lieber C.S., Jones D.P. and DeCarli L.M. (1965): *J. Clin. Invest.* 44: 1009-1021.
4. Iseri O.A., Lieber C.S. and Gottlieb L.S. (1966): *Am. J. Pathol.* 48: 535-555.
5. Yamada S., Mak K.M. and Lieber C.S. (1985): *Gastroenterology* 88: 1799-1806.
6. Cederbaum A.I., Lieber, C.S. and Rubin E. (1974): *Arch. Biochem. Biophys.* 165: 1187-1192.
7. Cederbaum A.I., Lieber, C.S. and Rubin E. (1976): *Arch. Biochem. Biophys.* 176: 525-538.
8. Cederbaum A.I., Lieber, C.S., Beattie D.S. and Rubin E. (1975): *J. Biol. Chem.* 250:5122-5129.
9. Matsuzaki S. and Lieber C.S. (1977): *Biochem. Biophys. Res. Commun.* 75: 1059-1065.
10. Tsukamoto H., French S.W., Benson, N., Delgado G., Rao G.A., Larkin E.C. and Largman C. (1985): *Hepatology* 5: 224-232.
11. Lieber C.S., DeCarli L.M. and Rubin E. (1975): *Proc. Natl. Acad. Sci. USA* 72:437-441.
12. Lieber C.S., Leo M.A., Mak K.M., DeCarli L.M. and Sato S. (1985): *Hepatology* 5: 561-572.
13. Lieber C.S., DeCarli L.M., Mak K.M., Kim C-I. and Leo M.A. (1990): *Hepatology* 12: 1390-1398.
14. Popper H. and Lieber C.S. (1980): *Am. J. Pathol.* 98: 695-716.
15. Lieber C.S. and Rubin E. (1968): *Am. J. Med.* 44: 200-206.
16. Lieber C.S. and Spritz N. (1966): *J. Clin. Invest.* 45: 1400-1411.
17. Rubin E. and Lieber C.S. (1968): *N. Engl. J. Med.* 278: 869-876.
18. Lane B.P. and Lieber C.S. (1966): *Am. J. Pathol.* 49: 593-603.
19. Lieber C.S. and DeCarli L.M. (1991): *J Hepatology* 12: 404-411.
20. Lieber C.S. (1990): *Alcohol Alcohol* 25: 157-176.
21. Lieber C.S. (1988): *Nutr. Rev.* 46: 241-245.
22. Lieber C.S. (1991): *Alcoholism: Clin. Exp. Res.* 15: 573-592.
23. Hernández-Muñoz R., Caballeria J., Baraona E., Uppal R., Greenstein R. and Lieber C.S. (1990): *Alcoholism: Clin. Exp. Res.* 14: 946-950.
24. Julkunen R.J.K., DiPadova C. and Lieber C.S. (1985): *Life Sci.* 37: 567-573.
25. Julkunen R.J.K., Tannenbaum L., Baraona E. and Lieber C.S. (1985): *Alcohol* 2: 437-441.
26. Caballeria J., Frezza M., Hernandez-Munoz R., DiPadova C., Korsten M.A., Baraona E. and Lieber C.S. (1989): *Gastroenterology* 97: 1205-1209.
27. DiPadova C., Worner T.M., Julkunen R.J.K. and Lieber C.S. (1987): *Gastroenterology* 92: 1169-1173.
28. Roine R., Gentry R.T., Hernández-Muñoz R., Baraona E. and Lieber C.S. (1990): *JAMA* 264: 2406-2408.
29. Caballeria J., Baraona E., Rodamilans M. and Lieber C.S. (1989): *Gastroenterology* 96: 388-392.
30. Roine R., DiPadova C., Frezza M., Hernández-Muñoz R., Baraona E. and Lieber C.S. (1990): *Gastroenterology* 98: 114 (abstract).
31. Frezza M., DiPadova C., Pozzato G., Terpin M., Baraona E. and Lieber C.S. (1990): *N. Engl. J. Med.* 322: 95-99.
32. Lieber C.S. and DeCarli L.M. (1968): *Science* 162: 917-918.
33. Lieber C.S. and DeCarli L.M. (1970): *J. Biol. Chem.* 245: 2505-2512.
34. Ohnishi K. and Lieber C.S. (1977): *J. Biol. Chem.* 252: 7124-7131.
35. Koop D.R., Morgan E.T., Tarr G.E. and Coon M.J. (1982): *J. Biol. Chem.* 257: 8472-8480.
36. Lasker J.M., Raucy J., Kubota S., Bloswick B.P., Black M. and Lieber C.S. (1987): *Biochem. Biophys. Res. Commun.* 148: 232-238.
37. Shaw S., Jayatilleke E., Ross W.A., Gordon E.R. and Lieber C.S. (1981): *J. Lab. Clin. Med.* 98: 417-425.

38. Lieber C.S., Casini A., DeCarli L.M., Kim C., Lowe N., Sasaki R. and Leo M.A. (1990): *Hepatology* 11: 165-172.
39. Savolainen E-R., Leo M.A., Timpl R. and Lieber C.S. (1984): *Gastroenterology* 87: 777-787.
40. Moshage H., Casini A. and Lieber C.S. (1990): *Hepatology* 12: 511-518.
41. Casini A., Cunningham M., Rojkind M. and Lieber C.S. (1991): *Hepatology* 13: 758-765.
42. Duce A.M., Ortiz P., Cabrero C. and Mato JM. (1988): *Hepatology* 8: 65-68.
43. Finkelstein J.D., Cello J.P. and Kyle W.E. (1974): *Biochem. Biophys. Res. Commun.* 61: 475-481.
44. Mato J.M. (1986): *Progress in protein-lipid interactions*. Vol. 2, pp. 267. Elsevier Scientific Publishing, New York.
45. Finkelstein J.D. and Martin J.J. (1986): *J. Biol. Chem.* 261: 1582-1587.
46. Hardwick D.F., Applegarth D.A., Cockcroft D.M., Ross P.M. and Cder R.J. (1970): *Metabolism* 19: 381-391.
47. Stramentinoli G., Gualano M. and Galli-Kienle M. (1979): *J. Pharmacol. Exp. Ther.* 209: 323-326.
48. Bombardieri G., Pappalardo G., Bernardi L., Barra D., Di Palma A. and Castrini G. (1983): *Int. J. Clin. Pharmacol. Ther. Toxicol.* 21: 186-188.
49. Hoffman D.R., Marion D.W., Cornatzer W.E. and Duerra JA. (1980): *J. Biol. Chem.* 255: 10822-10827.
50. Travers J., Varela J. and Mato J.M. (1984): *Biochem. Pharmacol.* 33: 1562-1564.
51. Engstrom M.A. and Benevenga N.J. (1987): *J. Nutr.* 117: 1820-1826.
52. Pezzoli C., Stramentinoli G., Galli-Kienele M. and Plaff E. (1978):. *Biochem. Biophys. Res. Commun.* 85: 1031-1038.
53. Zappia V., Galletti P. and Porcelli M. (1978): *FEBS Lett.* 90: 331-335.
54. Audubert F. and Vance D. (1983): *J. Biol. Chem.* 258: 10695-10701.
55. Quiram D.R. and Weinshilboum R.M. (1976): *J. Neurochemistry* 27: 1197-1203.
56. Giulidori P. and Stramentinoli G. (1984): *Anal. Biochem.* 137: 217-220.
57. Frezza M., Di Padova C. and the Italian Study Group for SAMe in Liver Disease. (1987): *Hepatology* 7: 1105 (abstract).
58. Okazaki I., Feinman L. and Lieber C.S. (1977): *Gastroenterology* 73: 1236.
59. Kato S., Murawaki Y. and Hirayama C. (1985): *Res Commun Chem Pathol Pharmacol* 47: 163-180.
60. Maruyama K., Feinman L., Fainsilber Z., Nakano M., Okazaki I. and Lieber C.S. (1982): *Life Sci.* 30: 1379-1384.
61. Lieber C.S., Li J-J., DeCarli L.M., Mak K.M., Kim C-I. and Leo M.A. (1990): *Hepatology* 4: 871 (abstract).
62. Orrego H., Blake J.E., Blendis L.M., Compton K.V. and Israel Y. (1987): *N. Engl. J. Med.* 317: 1421-1427.
63. Lieber C.S., Baraona E., Hernández-Muñoz R., Kubota S., Sato N., Kawano S., Matsumura T. and Inatomi N. (1989): *J. Clin. Invest.* 83: 1682-1690.
64. Kershenobich D., Vargas F., Garcia-Tsao G., Tomayo P.R., Gent M. and Rojkind M. (1988): *N. Engl. J. Med.* 318: 1709-1713.

Acknowledgements: Original studies summarized here were supported, in part, by DHHS grant AA03508, the Department of Veterans Affairs and the Kingsbridge Research Foundation.

LIVER FIBROGENESIS IN CHRONIC VIRAL AND ALCOHOLIC LIVER DISEASE

G.Annoni and B.Arosio

Fibrosis is only one of a constellation of histologic features that characterize viral and alcoholic liver disease and is one given particular consideration, because it represents a potentially irreversible form of injury, for which there is little available therapy (1). In the recent past, this specific area of investigation has significantly progressed and the molecular biology techniques are the basis for this terrific improvement (2).

In this chapter we discuss three points and in particular the cells implicated in the production of extracellular matrix, the soluble mediators responsible for their molecular modulation and finally the results of molecular biology studies in human liver pathology.

However, to short a very complex story, we will focus attention on one cell, the Ito cell, also known as hepatic lipocyte, perisinusoidal fat-storing cell or stellate cell and one soluble factor, TGF-β1.

On the basis of the immunohistochemical studies, Ito cells are considered to be one of the most important sites of the production of the extracellular matrix components (3).

This past year, we published a study on the molecular analysis of Ito cell gene expression, aimed at delineating the phenotype of these cells (4). Northern blot hybridization analysis comparing mRNA transcripts from freshly isolated Ito cells obtained from Sprogue-Dawley rats, and also from cells cultured for 7 days, showed that cultured Ito cells have a 17 times as much type I procollagen mRNA content, as freshly isolated cells, as determined by densitometry scanning.

The mRNA contents of type III and IV procollagen were 300% and 260% higher, in cultured cells than in freshly isolated cells, and the relative quantities of mRNAs for these collagens in cultured Ito cells were similar to those found in 3T3-L1 preadipocytes. Both cell types, cultured Ito cells and preadipocytes, contain primarily type I procollagen mRNA but also larger amounts of type III and IV procollagen mRNA, which is consistent with the biochemical observations of the increases in types I, III and IV collagen in cirrhosis.

In relation to the soluble mediators that may be implicated in hepatic fibroplasia, among the constellation of cytokines and growth factors, we have considered a family of proteins that are now commonly called TGF-β. These proteins have been discovered several times over the past decade and with each independent discovery a different function for the protein was identified (5). TGF-β is a homodimeric peptide with a molecular weight of 25 KD. The protein is produced by platelets, placental cells and many other cells.

D. Galmarini et al. (eds.), Drugs and the Liver: High Risk Patients and Transplantation, 119–124.

The mammalian TGF-β family consists of almost three related proteins, that recognize different receptors but that have overlapping activity. The genes and cDNAs for all the TGF-βs have been cloned and sequenced. A high degree of conservation - about 99% - between the human and the other mammalian TGF-β sequences, argues for a critical biological role of the protein across species. There are receptors for TGF-β on nearly all cells and the peptide is defined as a multifunctional regulator of cellular activity since it has opposite effects on different cells. In fact, TGF-β strongly inhibits the proliferation of normal and certain tumor-derived epithelial cells lines, including hepatocytes, but, in contrast, some mesenchymal cells proliferate at picomolar concentrations of the growth factor. TGF-β also has significant effects on connective tissue modulation.

We have investigated the role of TGF-β in liver fibrosis, employing both in vivo and in vitro experimental models (4, 6).

As the in vivo model, we adopted the toxin-induced injury of rats with CCl_4.

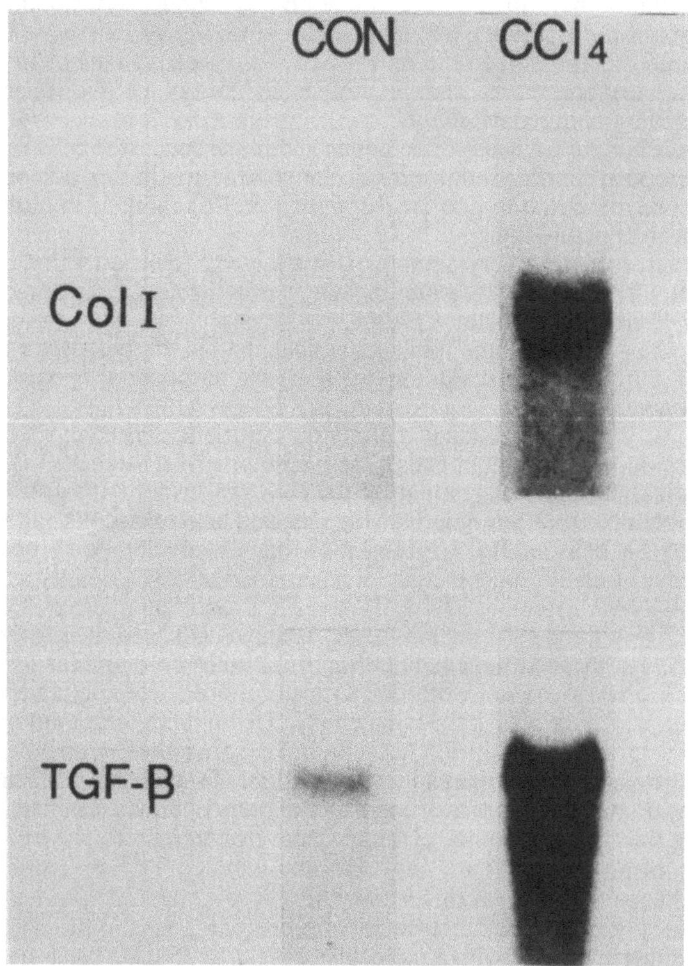

Fig. 1, Representative Northern blot hybridation study that identifies pro α1(I) collagen and TGF-β1 mRNA isolated from livers of control rats (CON) or CCl_4 treated rats (CCl_4).

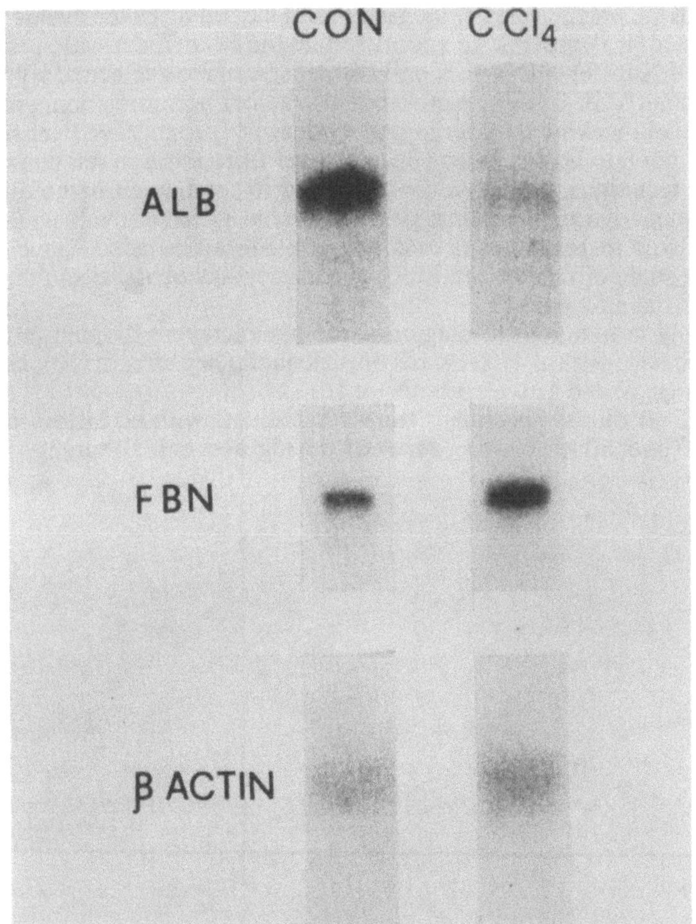

Fig. 2, Representative Northern blot hybridation study of total RNA isolated from livers of control rats (CON) compared with RNA from CCl_4 treated rats (CCl_4). RNA was hybridized with albumin, cellular fibronectin and β-actin probes.

After 8 weeks of treatment (Fig. 1), TGF-β1 mRNA steady state levels were significantly higher than in the controls, and the increase parallels that of pro α 2 (I) collagen. Interestingly (Fig. 2), at the same time albumin gene expression was reduced and expression of the gene coding for insoluble fibronectin was enhanced, again over that of control animals. To support a causal relationship between TGF-β1 and collagen synthesis, in vitro studies were also performed.For these, we studied the effects of TGF-β1 in Ito cells. Primary cultures of non-confluent Ito cells were treated with 0.1 nmol/L TGF-β1.

A greater than threefold increase in total collagen content was seen. Northern hybridization analysis of total RNA from these cells revealed a 280% increase in type I procollagen mRNA in TGF-β1 treated cells and, to our surprise, TGF-β1 treatment also led to increased production of TGF-β1 mRNA, thus suggesting an autocrine autostimulation of the Ito cells and a mechanism able to perpetuate the fibrogenic process.

Although the precise roles of the factors and the timing of the events remain to be determined, it is possible to speculate that the Ito cell activation is initiated by release of Kupffer cell factors or by direct stimulation of acetaldeyde or lactate. At this point TGF-β1 by paracrine but also autocrine stimulation, perpetuates the cell's activation, with the histological evidence of progressive liver fibrosis.

The last point to be discussed concerns liver fibroplasia in relation to molecular biology techniques that have been applied to the human pathology. In recent years we have examined this aspect and we have tried to evaluate the molecular mechanisms responsible for this process. In particular we have enrolled 30 patients; some of them with history of chronic alcohol abuse and the others with chronic viral infections (7).

According to histological diagnosis, the patients were divided in four groups: alcoholic hepatitis (n: 4), cirrhosis plus alcoholic hepatitis (n: 10), chronic active hepatitis (n: 6) and active cirrhosis (n: 10).

Wedge liver biopsy specimens from two patients with no history or laboratory signs of liver disease were obtained during abdominal surgery and used as controls.

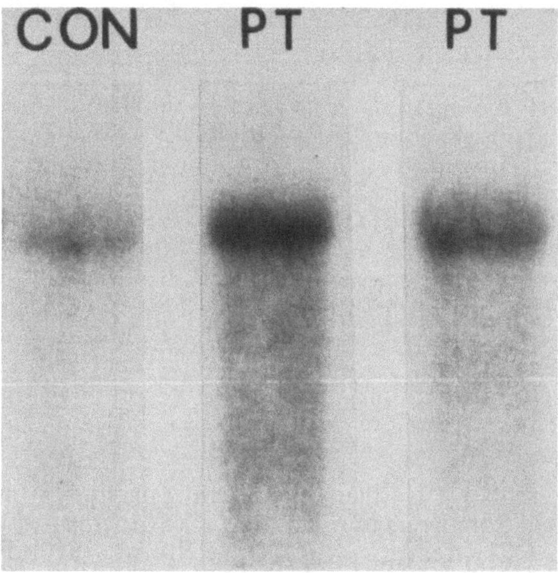

Fig. 3, Representative Northern blot hybridation study that identifies pro α1(I) -collagen mRNA in total RNA isolated from livers of controls (CON) or patients (PT).

The Fig. 3 shows a representative Northern Blot that identifies pro α^1 (I) collagen mRNA in a control and also in two patients with different degrees of histologically evaluated liver fibrosis. The cDNA for this assay was the human probe, HF 677. The densitometry scanning showed that all four groups of patients had higher procollagen mRNA levels than the controls, regardless of the ethiology of the disease or the presence of cirrhosis. These data clearly suggest that an increase in collagen synthesis may be a significant factor in the pathogenesis of hepatic fibrosis.

As we have just described, many data derived from in vitro and also in vivo experimental models strongly suggest a role of TGF β1 in liver fibroplasia.

Therefore, we attempted to define the role of TGF β1 in human hepatic fibrogenesis by examining expression of its gene and the correlation of this with type I collagen gene expression.

The Northern blot hybridization analysis for type I collagen and TGF β1 revealed increased levels of expression of both genes as determined by the densitometry scans of all the blots and also a significant correlation between TGF β1 and collagen type I mRNA levels.

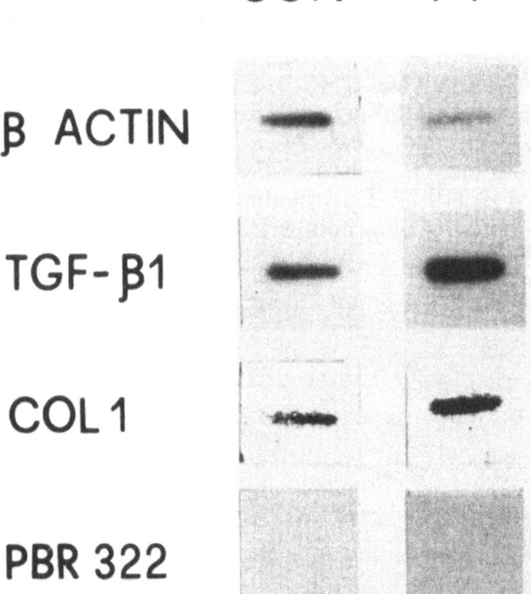

Fig. 4, Representative nuclear run-on assay analyzing the transcriptional rates of TGF-β1 and pro α1(I) collagen genes from a liver of a control patient (CON) compared to a patient with fibrotic liver disease (PT).

In an attempt to determine more precisely the level of gene regulation responsible for this increase in the steady state mRNA levels of TGF β1, we employed the nuclear run-on assay to analyse transcriptional rates (8). The Fig. 4 is a representative nuclear run-on assay clearly demonstrating an increase in the transcriptional rate of TGF β1 gene in a patient with liver disease over that of control. Taking all the results together, we can therefore summarize:

1) We have found an increase in steady state type I collagen mRNA levels;
2) similar results were also found for TGF β1 and for it, an increase in the transcription rate of the gene could be responsible for the high steady state mRNA levels;
3) finally, there seems to be a correlation between the TGF β1 and type I collagen gene.

The results discussed here represent only the beginning of the possibilities for application of molecular biology to the study of human liver fibrosis.

In particular, possible future areas of investigation might include identification by in situ hybridization of the specific cell type(s) responsible for collagen synthesis and the definition of the roles of some cytokines and growth factors in the disease evolution.

REFERENCES

1. Berk P.D., Editor (1990): Connective Tissue Metabolism and Hepatic Fibrosis. Thieme Medical Publishers, Inc, New York.
2. Zern M.A., Wheiner F.R., Creja M.J., Degli Esposti S., (1990): In: Molecular Biology, edited by Mc Graw-Hill Book Company.
3. Clément B., Emonard E., Russel M., (1984): Cell Mol. Biol. 30: 489-496.
4. Weiner F.R., Giambone M.A., Creja M.J., Shah A., Amowy G., Zern M.A. (1990): Hepatology, 11: 111-117.
5. Messagué M.J. (1987): Cell, 49: 437-438.
6. Creja M.J., Wheiner F.R., Flenders K.C., Zern M.A. (1989): J. Cell. Biol., 108: 2477-2482.
7. Annoni G., Wheiner F.R., Colombo M., Creja M.J., Zern M.A. (1990): Gastroenterology, 98: 197-202.
8. Annoni G., Wheiner F.R., Zern M.A. (1991): Journal of Hepatology, in press.

HEPATOCELLULAR CARCINOMA

A.Sangiovanni, M.G.Rumi, G.Covini and M.Colombo

Introduction

Hepatocellular carcinoma (HCC) is a highly malignant tumor with an exremely poor prognosis and with an incidence estimated to be at least 250,000 cases per year, worldwide[1]. In recent years epidemiological surveys, molecular biology studies and prospective investigations of certain groups of patients have greatly improved our understanding of the etiology, pathogenesis and natural history of this cancer. In this paper, we review currently available data on the role of hepatitis viruses and alcohol in human hepatocarcinogenesis.

Hepatitis B virus

The association between hepatitis B virus (HBV) and HCC appears to be strong, specific and consistent[2,3]. The prevalence of HBsAg is common in the areas of the world in which there is also a high incidence of liver cancer. In a prospective study of 22,707 Chinese men in Taiwan, Beasley (3) found that the incidence of the tumor in the HBsAg positive population was 473/100,000 persons per year, compared to only 4.6 in the HBsAg negative individuals (relative risk = 102). Another important piece of evidence connecting HCC to HBV comes from the study of either naturally or

D. Galmarini et al. (eds.), Drugs and the Liver: High Risk Patients and Transplantation, 125–130.

experimentally infected woodchucks. Ninety-seven percent of captive animals infected at birth with woodchuck hepatitis virus (WHV) and maintained in captivity developed HCC after 17-36 months of persistent infection. The time of life when the infection occurs is important for subsequent development of the tumor. Infection early in life or during pregnancy frequently becomes persistent and frequently results in HCC, probably acting in conjunction with additional family-related factors. Infection with HBV in adults carries a far lower risk of a carrier state developing and of subsequent HCC development. No single mechanism has been proposed for HBV-induced oncogenesis, and most data point against the existence of a viral transforming oncogene. One general mechanism by which HBV acts as a carcinogenic agent is its integration into the host cellular genome[4]. The persistence of viral integrations in susceptible animals and in man may cause genetic alterations and epigenetic phenomena. The unstable nature of cellular DNA into which hepadnavirus has been integrated may cause such chromosome alterations as deletions of cellular DNA, transformation and duplication of viral and cellular DNA and the chromosomal translocations that are found in HCC. The gradual accumulation of these mutations in the cellular genome may predispose a cell to malignant transformation. More specific mechanisms of genetic damage such as insertional mutagenesis and transactivation, have also been observed in man and animals where virus integrations have created new genes with potential regulatory properties. In livers in which no viral insertions are found HCC may also be the result of the inactivation of tumor suppressor genes. Recently, point mutations in the suppressor p53 gene (mutational hotspots) have been identified in some HCC from Chinese and South African patients living in areas endemic for HBV and aflatoxin[5,6]. Gene mutations consisted preferentially in guanin to thymidin substitutions within clustering at codon 249. The presence of this hotspot in HCC implies that there is a selective advantage for these specific mutations that could be etiopathogenetically important. In fact, in appropriate experimental conditions, aflatoxin

B1,may cause similar mutations and HBV, which is also implicated in HCC in Africa and China, could interact through a virally-induced protein with the specific mutant p 53. Thus, the oncogenic role of HBV seems to be particularly important in most Asian and African countries where high HBV endemicity is mantained by infection occurring early in life, but not in the Western world and Japan where this tumor is often related to other factors such as alcohol and hepatitis C.

Hepatitis C virus

Several types of evidence connect HCC with the RNA hepatitis C virus (HCV)[7]. In the last decade in Japan, the number of HCC associated with HBV has decreased by 50% while that of HBsAg-negative tumors in patients with history of blood transfusions has increased, suggesting that HCV has a leading role in the etiology of this tumor. Sequential development of cirrhosis and HCC has been observed in patients with transfusion-associated and community-acquired hepatitis. Development of chronic non-A non-B hepatitis was also observed in one chimpanzee which was experimentally infected with human plasma, with subsequent development of HCC 6 years after the infection. Finally, a high prevalence of serum antibody to HCV has been observed in patients with HCC, particularly in the HBsAg-negative subgroup of patients[8]. Interestingly, nearly all of the HCV infected patients had cirrhosis, whereas a consistent number of them also had other risk factors, such as HBsAg and history of alcohol abuse, indicating that in many patients both cirrhosis and HCC may have multifactorial origins. In some patients, RNA sequences of HCV were isolated from the tumor tissue by the polymerase chain reaction. Although these findings establish a strong link between chronic HCV infection and neoplastic transformation of the liver, it is unlikely that HCV plays a direct role in HCC, since no reverse transcriptase activity has been found in infected liver tissue. One current opinion is that HCV rather than having a direct oncogenic effect, promotes HCC through cirrhosis which is per se an important risk factor for this tumor.

Alcohol

An association between ethanol and human HCC is biologically plausible, since HCC has been observed in 5-20% of all cases of micronodular cirrhosis and alcohol promotes cancer in such organs as the oral cavity, pharynx, larynx and esophagus[9]. Although ethanol has not been shown experimentally to be mutagenic, it might have effects on DNA metabolism that could be associated with carcinogenic activity. Acetaldehyde, the first metabolite of ethanol, can induce sister chromatid exchanges in hamster ovary cells grown in tissue cultures. Moreover, ethanol-fed animals have prolonged persistence of DNA adducts, which signals reduced capacity of the cell to repair DNA damage. The association of alcohol abuse with human HCC has been investigated in 22 studies involving more than 2,700 patients: it was present in 14 studies (relative risk:1.3-12.0) but not in the remaining 8[10]. Alcohol had a dose-dependent effect, with approximately a 40% excess HCC risk entailed by heavy consumption. However, case-control studies in which drinking patterns are ascertained subsequent to HCC diagnosis could be biased by the patient's tendency to underreport alcohol consumption. In areas where the prevalence of HBV carriers is low, alcohol may be an important factor for HCC: it does promote liver cirrhosis, the development and progression of which may act in conjunction with other enviromental liver carcinogens. One study in Japan demonstrated that development of HCC occurred 10 years earlier in alcoholic patients who were HBsAg carriers compared to non carriers[11].

Cirrhosis

The above studies indicate that patients with cirrhosis are a risk population for HCC. In fact, 30-40% of patients who died of cirrhosis were found on autopsy to have HCC, and 90% of patients with HCC have associated cirrhosis[12]. Close follow-up studies of cirrhotic patients with highly sensitive and specific diagnostic methods, such as real-time ultrasound, have led to recognition of the tumor at an early stage[13]. The significance of the association of HCC and cirrhosis is still obscure and no single explanation accounts for the various forms the association between cirrhosis and HCC takes in different parts of the world. In some patients HCC could be the inevitable consequence of long-standing hepatic disease whilst in others it could be an independent response to a hepatic insult common to HCC and cirrhosis. A key factor in the pathogenesis of HCC developing in patients with cirrhosis is liver cell regeneration. Cell regeneration during cirrhosis, unlike that occurring in normal livers, may be oncogenic since it is associated with abnormal hormone patterns, alteration in the liver array of parenchymal cells, altered production of growth factors and abnormal oncogene expressions.

Conclusions

Whatever is the biological meaning of the association between HCC, and cirrhosis, such an association provides a formidable means for prospectively studying patients who are at risk of HCC. Early diagnosis of HCC is possible not only due to the knowledge of the risk factors for this tumor, but also because HCC has a very long phase of intrahepatic growth and tends to grow as a solitary mass. Early diagnosis is also possible because sensitive and relatively inexpensive diagnostic tools are available. Recently, in a consensus development conference held in Milan (Italy) chronic carriers of HBsAg and patients with cirrhosis were identified as high risk patients for HCC and therefore as candidates for periodic screening[14]. It was recommended that healthy HBsAg carriers have yearly determinaton of serum alphafetoprotein (AFP) and ALT, and patients with cirrhosis be screened every 6 months by abdominal ultrasouds and AFP. Several prospective studies of Italian patients with cirrhosis now in progress have led to the identification of many patients with small tumors. Studies are in progress to assess whether early diagnosis of HCC may also increase the number of operable patients and reduce the mortality rate for this tumor.

References

1. Parkin D.M., Muir C.S. (1984): Bull.W.H.O., 62:163-182.
2. Popper H. (1988): In: Viral Hepatitis and Liver Disease, edited by Zuckerman A.J. pp. 719-722. Alan R. Liss, New York.
3. Beasley R.P. (1987): Cancer, 61: 1842-1856.
4. Rogler C.E. (1990): Cancer Cell-Mon. Rev., 2: 366-370.
5. Hsu I.C., Metcalf R.A., Sun T., Welsh J.A., Wang N.J., Harris C.C. (1991): Nature, 350: 427-428.
6. Bressac B., Kew M., Wands J., Ozturk M. (1991): Nature, 350: 429-431.
7. Tabor E. (1990): J. Med. Virol., 335: 300-301.
8. Colombo M., Kuo G., Choo Q.L., Donato M.F., Del Ninno E., Tommasini M.A., Dioguardi N., Houghton M. (1989): Lancet, 2: 1006-1009.
9. Lieber C.S., Garro A., Leo M.A., Mak K.M., Worner T. (1986): Hepatology, 6: 1005-1019.
10. Austin H. (1991): In: Etiology Pathology and Treatment of Hepatocellular Carcinoma in North America, edited by E. Tabor, A.M. Di Bisceglie, R.H. Purcell pp. 35-56. Gulf Publishing Company, Houston.
11. Ohnishi K., Iida S., Iwama S., Goto N., Nomura F., Takashi M., Okuda K. (1982): Cancer, 49: 672-677.
12. Kew M.C., Popper H. (1984): Semin. Liver Dis., 4: 136-146.
13. Colombo M., de Franchis R., Del Ninno E., Sangiovanni A., De Fazio C., Tommasini M., Donato M.F., Piva A., Di Carlo V., Dioguardi N. N. Engl. J. Med. (in press)
14. Colombo M. J. Hepatology (in press)

TREATMENT OF IRON DEPENDENT CHRONIC LIVER DISEASE

G. Fiorelli , A. Piperno, A.L. Fracanzani, M.D. Cappellini , R. Romano, R. D'Alba and S. Fargion

IRON AND LIVER DAMAGE

In man, several disorders can lead to excess tissue iron deposition, including genetic hemochromatosis (GH) and the various causes of secondary hemochromatosis that is chronic transfusion dependent anemias, sideroblastic anemia, alcoholic cirrhosis and porphyria cutanea tarda (PCT) (1). In all these conditions liver damage is a common finding. Clinical and experimental data indicate that iron is involved in the pathogenesis of hepatic fibrosis, cirrhosis and consequently hepatocellular carcinoma (HCC). GH which is a hereditary disease characterized by severe iron overload and which is much more common than was originally thought (about 1 in 220 white Northern Europeans is affected (2)), can be considered as a representative model of iron induced liver disease. Whereas the role of iron is clear in GH, in PCT and iron loading anemia it is less clear whether iron acts as a cofactor in the pathogenesis of liver damage in other conditions as chronic alcoholic and viral liver diseases.

Clinical data

The best evidence that iron is responsible for liver damage in patients with GH derives from the observation that early diagnosis and phlebotomy therapy result in a significantly longer survival (3) and that the development of fibrosis and cirrhosis depends on a combination of factors including hepatic iron concentration and the lenght of time that the liver has been exposed to the high iron concentration. A threshold value has also been demonstrated for the occurrence of cirrhosis: in absence of hepatotoxic cofactors such as alcoholism, 22 mg of iron/g dry tissue have to be accumulated in

D. Galmarini et al. (eds.), Drugs and the Liver: High Risk Patients and Transplantation, 131–136.

the liver (4). This relation between the degree of iron overload and liver damage is also shown by the finding that our GH patients who had an early diagnosis were iron depleted by removing less than 10 g whereas in fibrotic or cirrhotic patients the total iron removed was much higher. In contrast, when chronic alcohol abuse or chronic hepatitis viral infection coexisted with GH, the amount of iron removed was lower than 10 g, also in patients with cirrhosis. Thus iron and alcohol or hepatitis virus infection can be synergistic in causing liver damage.

Experimental data and physiopathology

Despite the varied clinical evidence for liver injury as a consequence of iron overload, the specific pathophysiological mechanisms for hepatocellular injury, fibrosis, cirrhosis and carcinoma are poorly understood. The most likely unifying mechanism is one that involves an iron-induced peroxidative injury to phospholipids of organelle membranes (5). However, the form of intracellular iron responsible for initiating the peroxidative cascade is unknown. It is possible that in presence of severe iron overload the iron carrier molecules are overwhelmed, and iron may decompartmentalize, reaching sites to which it normally does not have access (6). In fact, it is believed that a non-heme, non-storage iron protein exists within cells, loosely bound to low molecular weight compounds, amino acids and nucleotides. This iron fraction probably causes cell injury and death, damaging cellular lysosomes, and mitochondrial and microsomal membranes (5). Fibrosis can develop after these processes, but, it has been demonstrated that iron is able, by itself, to induce hepatic fibrosis. An increase in collagen fibrils, hepatic hydroxyproline content and hepatic prolyl hydroxylase activity has been reported in iron overloaded rats (7). On the basis of these data it was postulated that excess iron provides a direct stimulus to collagen biosynthesis, without prior iron mediated cellular injury. This was further confirmed by evidence that iron can increase α 2 collagen m RNA in rat liver (8).

Iron and hepatocellular carcinoma

Based on the observation that most patients with cirrhotic GH die of HCC, it was suggested that iron can be carcinogenic. In addition, several reports have indicated a relation between increased iron body stores and risk of cancer (9,10). Experimental data support the hypothesis that decompartmentalized iron and/or free radicals can interact with DNA with consequent mutations and chromosomal aberrations (11). In addition, an activation of proto-oncogenes c-fos and c-myc in mouse epidermal cells has been shown after iron-induced oxidant stress (12).

Our data on Italian patients with GH confirm the high risk of HCC and indicate that HCC always occurs in a cirrhotic liver (3). Thus although cirrhosis appears to be a *sine qua non,* iron may exert its carcinogenic role interacting directly with DNA and giving rise through the years to a clone of mutated cells which in a cirrhotic liver are more prone to proliferate in a disorganized fashion. In addition, the high prevalence of hepatitis B (HBV) and C (HCV) virus infection in our population of patients with GH supports the observation that iron and virus play a synergistic role in the pathogenesis of HCC, as demonstrated by the lower amount of iron removed up to depletion in HBV or HCV positive patients who developed HCC with respect to those without virus infection (13). This could also happen in patients with chronic non-GH liver disease and iron overload; several data support the hypothesis that iron can facilitate the persistence of HBV and probably also HCV infection (13,14).

Thus, iron removal therapy is indicated not only in GH but also in chronic liver diseases in which iron overload coexists.

IRON DEPLETION THERAPY

Considering that iron is the causative agent in the development of liver damage in patients with iron overload, therapy needs to be aimed at the complete removal of iron not only to ameliorate iron induced damage but also to prevent it.

Iron overload is treated mainly by: phlebotomy and chelation .

Phlebotomy

Phlebotomy is usually performed in GH and PCT. Patients undergo weekly or biweekly removal of 400-500 ml of blood with which is removed 200-250 mg of iron, until iron depletion is achieved (serum ferritin below 20 µg/l). Afterwards maintenance therapy consists of removal of 400-500 ml of blood every 2-3 months (1). In patients with GH the duration of therapy varies; the earlier it is started, the shorter it is. However, it has been reported that iron depletion therapy lasting more than 18 months is a negative prognostic factor (3). In contrast, patients with PCT seldom need more than 10-15 phlebotomies.

Phlebotomy is usually very well tolerated in GH patients, unless cardiomyopathy or severe cirrhosis is present. When phlebotomy cannot be performed due to the poor clinical condition of the patients, the therapy is based on iron chelating agents.

Chelation therapy

Chelating agents are the only available treatment for iron loading anemias.

Desferrioxamine

Desferrioxamine (DF) is currently the most clinically useful iron chelator available, administrable only by parenteral routes (subcutaneous or intravenous infusion of 20-80 mg/Kg daily several days a week) (15). A high dose intravenous treatment (6-12 g of DF daily for 12 hours) has been proposed for patients whose compliance with treatment is poor, who fail to establish a negative iron balance and whose rate of iron removal with subcutaneous infusion of DF may be too slow to prevent severe organ damage and early death (15). The major problems related to DF are the cumbersome mode of parenteral administration which results in poor compliance in adolescents and adults, serious toxicity with intensive use, and high cost. Visual and audiologic abnormalities are the most frequently reported toxic effects of DF. Whether toxicity is related to drug dose and degree of iron overload and whether other factors are involved in the pathogenesis of visual and hearing disorders during DF chelation are still controversial (16). For these reasons the most urgent need of patients with transfusional iron loading anemia is an effective, safe, inexpensive **oral** iron chelator.

Oral chelators

Various studies have been performed in the last few years on oral iron chelators. Although many new compounds have been tested *in vitro* and *in vivo* in animals, until now the only oral chelator currently under clinical trial is 1,2-dimethyl-3-hydroxypyrid-4-one (L1).

Over 180 patients and volunteers have received L1 in the UK, India, Italy, the Netherlands, Switzerland and Canada. L1 was effective in increasing urinary iron excretion in all transfusional iron loaded patients. The amount of iron excreted was comparable to that obtained by DF (17). Toxicity testing of L1 and relative compounds has produced apparently discrepant findings (17,18). The adverse effects reported were musculoskeletal pains, agranulocytosis in a Blackfan Diamond patient, and gastric intolerance (17). Of the patients treated two died soon after stopping L1, one with thalassemia in a very advanced stage of the disease and one with a myelodysplastic syndrome. It is not easy to relate these deaths to administration of the drug (19).

Although L1 is being given in several centers, its suitability for clinical trials has been debated and some authors suggest that its use as a therapeutic alternative to subcutaneous DF cannot yet be recommended (18).

Efficacy of iron depletion therapy

The beneficial effects of iron depletion in patients with thalassemia major was demonstrated by Ridson et al. (20). They observed that nontreated patients showed a marked and progressive increase of liver fibrosis unlike the treated patients who presented no significant change in the degree of fibrosis. These data have been confirmed by more recent studies on patients with GH who showed a significant reduction of the degree of hepatic fibrosis, evaluated by morphometric studies, and a decrease of the hepatocyte lysosome volume density after treatment (21,22).

Depletion therapy also influences biochemical variables. After iron removal we observed a significant decrease of serum alanine transferase (ALT) (80.4 $\pm$ 43.6 vs 38.8 $\pm$ 18.2 UI/L) in 52 patients with GH and a decrease of urinary porphyrin (5500 $\pm$ 1620 vs 350 $\pm$ 48 µg/l) in 50 patients with PCT.

The benefits of iron depletion therapy have been established by different studies demonstrating that cirrhotic patients with GH and patients with thalassemia major treated by phlebotomy or chelation therapy have significantly longer survival (3,15).

New prospects in the use of iron chelators

Because of the crucial role of iron in the generation of toxic oxygen products, new therapeutic applications for iron chelators have emerged in these last years since oxygen radical mediated tissue damage is involved in many pathological conditions.

DF is able to decrease hydroxyl radical production as demonstrated in animal and human models (23). The synthesis of HBV surface antigen by PLC/CRF/5 human hepatoma cells as well as HBV virion production by hepatoma Hep G2 cells was inhibited by the addition of DF to the tissue culture media (24). Recent studies have shown that DF inhibits *in vitro* replication of HIV-1 being able to reduce viral p24 antigen expression and reverse transcriptase activity and the levels of *gag* and *env* genes in cell cultures (25,26). These data suggest that DF might interfere with viral replication possibly by inhibiting iron-dependent ribonucleotide reductase.

Anti tumor activity of DF has been observed in liver cancer cells *in vitro* and *in vivo* in athymic nude mice (27,28). By removing iron, DF apparently inhibits the first step of DNA synthesis of the tumor cells. On the basis of these results it has been suggested that DF may have a place in anticancer regimens in combination with other agents for the treatment of patients with HCC (27,28).

Investigation should clarify whether iron chelators, old and news may be useful alone or in combination therapy in liver pathology in which iron seems not to be the *primum movens* of the disease.

References

1. Halliday J.W., Powell L.W. (1982): Sem. Haematol., 19:42-45
2. Edwards C.Q., Griffen L.M., Goldard D., Drummond C., Skalnick M.H., Kushner J.P.(1988): N. Engl. J. Med., 318:1355-1362.

3. Niederau C., Fisher R., Sonnemberg A., Stremmel W., Trampisch H.J., Strohmeyer J. (1985): N. Engl. J. Med., 313: 1252-1262.
4. Basset M.L., Halliday J.W., Powell L.W. (1986): Hepatology, 6: 24-29.
5. Bacon B.R., Britton R.S. (1990): Hepatology, 11:123-137.
6. Mulligan M., Althouse B., Linder M.C. (1986): Int. J. Biochem., 18:791-798.
7. Weintraub L.R., Goral A., Grasso J., Granzblau C., Sulliwan A., Sulliwan S. (1985): Br. J. Haematol., 59:321-331.
8. Pietrangelo A., Rocchi E., Schiaffonati L., Ventura E., Cairo G. (1990): Hepatology, 11:798-804.
9. Stevens R.J., Johns Y., Micozzi M.S., Taylor P.R. (1988): N. Engl. J. Med., 319:1047-1052.
10. Selby J.V., Friedman G.D. (1988): Int. J. Cancer, 41: 677-682.
11. Loeb L.A., James E.A., Weltersdorph A.M., Klebanoff S.J. (1988): Proc. Natl. Acad. Sci. USA, 85:3918-3922.
12. Crawford D., Zbinden I., Amstad P., Cerutti P. (1988): Oncogene, 3: 27-32.
13. Fargion S., Piperno A., Fracanzani A.L., Cappellini M.D., Romano R., Fiorelli G. (1991): It. J. Gastroenterol., 23 (in press).
14. Piperno A., D'Alba R., Roffi L., Pozzi M., Farina A., Vecchi L., Fiorelli G. (1991): Arch. Virol., (in press).
15. Cohen A.(1990): Sem. Haematol., 27: 86-90.
16. Olivieri N.F., Buncic J.R., Chew E., Gallant T., Harrison R.W., Keenan L., Logan W., Mitchell D., Ricci G., Skarf B., Tailor M., Freedman M.H. (1986): N. Engl. J. Med., 314:869-873.
17. Kontoghiorghes G.S. (1991) Eur. J. Clin. Invest., 21:57
18. Olivieri N.F., Koren G., Hermann C., Bentur Y., Chung D., Klein J., St. Louis P., Freedman M.H., Mc Clelland R.A., Tempton D.M. (1990): Lancet, 336: 1275-1279.
19. Editorial. (1989): Lancett, ii: 1016-1017.
20. Ridson R.A., Barry M., Flynn D. (1974) Am. J. Pathol 116: 83-95.
21. Le Sage C.D., Baldus W.P., Green J.F. (1989): Hepatology, 10: 575.
22. Stal P., Glaumann H., Hultcrantz R. (1990): J.Hepathol., 11: 172-180.
23. Weimberg K. (1990): Am. J. Pedriat. Haematol. Onc., 12: 9-13.
24. Schwartz K.B., Korba B.(1990): Hepatology, 12:972.
25. Tabor E., Epstein J.S., Hewlett I.K., Lee S.F. (1991): Lancet, 337:795.
26. Baruchel S., Gao Q., Wainberg M.A. (1991): Lancet, 337:1350.
27. Hann H.W.L., Stahlhut M.W., Hann C.L. (1990) Hepatology, 11:566-569.
28. Hann H.W.L., Stahlhut M.W., Maddrey W.C. (1990): Hepatology, 12:912.

LIVER TRANSPLANTATION FOR CHRONIC LIVER DISEASE

David H. Van Thiel, M.D.

Liver transplantation as a clinical procedure has advanced considerably since its introduction in 1963 (1). The procedure no longer is considered intrinsically news worthy and is being performed worldwide at an increasing number of locations. Moreover, at some hospitals it is being performed several times a day and at others it is a routinely scheduled surgical procedure. With these changes in the frequency of performance of the procedure and the number of locations at which the procedure is being performed, the indications for the procedure have changed also. The procedure is still being performed as a life saving procedure for those with far advanced chronic liver disease but the basic rationale for the procedure has changed from one of a desperate effort at life salvage to one of preservation of life with an improvement in the quality of the preserved life and potentially also a cure of the underlying hepatic disease (2,3).

Currently, the performance of a liver transplant for chronic liver disease is expected to achieve a 5 year survival that is between 75-95%. Moreover, survivors are expected to be able to return to their work, raise families and assume all of the pleasures and responsibilities of their extended life. On the other hand, a cure of their liver disease occurs in some cases but not all and frequently one liver disease is traded for another such as one due to a biliary or vascular complication of the surgical procedure or an immunologically mediated response to the allograft (4,6).

Table 1 shows a listing of types of chronic liver disease for which liver transplantation has been performed. Two of the more common indications for liver transplantation worldwide are particularly common in

D. Galmarini et al. (eds.), Drugs and the Liver: High Risk Patients and Transplantation, 137–142.

Italy. These are liver transplantation for viral liver disease and neoplastic liver disease.

TABLE 1. Chronic Liver Disease and Orthotopic Liver Transplantation

1) viral liver disease	6) toxic induced liver disease
2) neoplastic liver disease	7) congenital-developmental liver disease
3) metabolic liver disease	8) trauma
4) cholestatic liver disease	9) vascular liver disease
5) autoimmune liver disease	

Liver transplantation for viral liver disease can be performed for either acute fulminant or subfulminant liver disease due to any of a large number of viruses or for chronic viral liver disease (2,3). In the latter case, hepatitis B, hepatitis B + hepatitis D, hepatitis C and the newly identifiable hepatitis non A, non B, non C are the principal indications for OLTx. Often a given recipient may have evidence for prior viral hepatitis due to 2 or more of the above listed viral liver diseases. Nonetheless, the particular viral disease necessitating transplantation in a given case can be determined based upon the identification of specific viral antigens or nucleic acids in liver cells, serum or circulating mononuclear cells of the proposed recipient. Unfortunately, recurrent viral liver disease rather than a cure is common when viral hepatitis is the indication for OLTx (7,8). Recurrent hepatitis B is almost universal in those who are HBV-DNA positive prior to transplantation. It is also very likely to occur (80% of cases) in those who are HBeAg+ who are HBV-DNA negative by current assay techniques. Worse yet, it can occur in recipients who are HBV-DNA negative and HBsAb positive prior to OLTx in some cases. Disease recurrence when it occurs takes on a virulent course and can run the full spectrum of viral liver disease from acute hepatitis to cirrhosis or even cirrhosis with hepatic cancer in as short a time as 2 or 3 years (7,8). Worse yet, should re-transplantation be offered, with each subsequent transplant the natural history of the liver disease is halved (8).

Not all is grim, however. Several groups have reported that the use of active and passive immunization particularly in cases that are HBV-DNA negative and HBeAg negative prior to transplantation can eliminate disease recurrence as long as the use of passive immunization is practiced (9,10).

The situation appears to be less bad with chronic

HCV with disease recurrence occurring in 10-30% of cases post-transplantation (11). The long term prognosis for the cases with disease recurrence, however, is as yet uncertain. Children with recurrent HCV disease particularly those transplanted urgently for fulminant non A, non B hepatitis appear to be uniquely at risk to develop aplastic anemia in the immediate post-transplant period (12). In such cases, this complication determines the outcome.

The prognosis for those with recurrent non A, non B, non C disease is currently uncertain as this disease has only recently been identifiable with the development of assays for the detection of HCV.

Interferon therapy for chronic hepatitis has been shown to be useful and is gaining increasing acceptance (13). The situation is the same for liver graft recipients (14). The experience to date with interferon therapy for viral hepatitis has shown that the use of the agent prior to OLTx is difficult and dangerous and can precipitate hepatic failure or cause lethal sepsis (15). The use of the drug peri-operatively is also difficult but can be accomplished (16). The most experience has been with the use of interferon in cases of clinically evident disease recurrence in the post-operative period (14). The use of interferon post-operatively is associated with remissions of disease due to hepatitis non A, non B, non C and hepatitis C and rarely also HBV. Partial remissions being defined as a greater than 50% reduction in liver enzymes with treatment occurs in cases of hepatitis non A, non B, non C > hepatitis B > hepatitis C.

TABLE 2. Neoplastic liver disease and OLTx

Benign	Malignant
multiple adenoma	fibrolamellar
hemangioma	hepatocellular
	hemangioendothelioma
	neuroendocrine tumors
	cholangiolar carcinoma
	unusual tumors

The indications for liver transplantation for neoplastic disease are shown in Table 2. Obviously the prognosis is best for those with benign tumors and cures are to be expected in such cases. In contrast, cures can be expected in only 25-30% of those transplanted for malignant disease. The disease free interval prior to the detection of recurrent disease determines the long term prognosis of those transplanted for malignant disease and is greatest for those with tumors such as hemangioendothelioma and fibrolamellar tumors and shorter for those with cholangiolar and the more usual forms of hepatocellular carcinoma (17). Nonetheless, it must be pointed out that liver transplantation for malignant disease is applied only to cases that are not otherwise resectable and typically in cases with far advanced disease. For such individuals, survival beyond 6 months or a year without transplantation is rarely if ever obtainable. Thus liver transplantation, although marred by disease recurrence in most cases, is the only hope and can produce cures in as many as a quarter or third of cases (18). Most importantly, particularly for those with disease recurrence, the quality of life extended by OLTx is good. As a result, liver transplantation for hepatic cancer is the best available form of disease treatment in terms of life quality without intent to cure.

Finally, liver transplantation for chronic cholestatic liver disease is a major indication for the procedure both in Italy and worldwide (18,19). Moreover, the results with liver transplantation for these indications are among the best achievable with 5 year survival rates of 80-95%. The specific indications for liver transplantation for chronic cholestatic liver disease include endstage disease, portal hypertension with variceal bleeding, hepatic osteodystrophy, and intractable pruritus. The procedure should be applied before the underlying liver disease leads to the development of thoracic cage boney involvement as the presence for such disease adversely affects the post-operative course particularly that which occurs in the ICU.

It goes without saying that ideally, liver transplantation should be offered to those with primary sclerosing cholangitis before the disease is complicated by cholangiolar carcinoma which currently is seen in 10% of the cases receiving a liver transplant or colonic adenocarcinoma which can occur in those with underlying ulcerative colitis (19,20). Moreover, those recipients of liver transplantation with ulcerative colitis need to be followed closely post-operatively for the development of colonic carcinoma (20). In such cases, annual colonoscopy is indicated.

Liver transplantation for chronic liver disease beyond these three indications is performed frequently for indications such as those identified in Table 1 but less often than for those identified above and with highly variable results. Nonetheless, liver transplantation for chronic liver disease of all types is widely accepted and has dramatically changed the face of hepatology both as a clinical science and a medical subspecialty.

REFERENCES

1. Starzl T.E., Marchioro T.L., Von Kaulla K.N., Hermann G., Brittain R.S., Waddell W.R. (1963): Surg. Gynecol. Obstet., 117:659-676.
2. Starzl T.E., Demetris A.J., Van Thiel D.H. (1989): N. Engl. J. Med., 321:1014-1022.
3. Starzl T.E., Demetris A.J., Van Thiel D.H. (1989): N. Engl. J. Med., 321:1092-1099.
4. Lerut J.P., Gordon R.D., Tzakis A.G., Stieber A.C., Iwatsuki S., Starzl T.E. (1988): Helf. Chir. Acta., 55:367-378.
5. Lerut J.P., Demetris A.J., Stieber A.C., Marsh J.W., Gordon R.D., Esquivel C.O., Iwatsuki S., Starzl T.E. (1988): Transplant International 1:127-130.
6. Wight D.G.D., Portmann B. (1987): In: Liver Transplantation, edited by R.Y. Calne pp. 385-435. Greene & Stratton, New York.
7. Demetris A.J., Todo S., Van Thiel D.H., Fung J.J., Sysn G., Ming W., Kakizoe S., Starzl T.E. (1990): Am. J. Pathol., 137:667-676.
8. Todo S., Demetris A.J., Van Thiel D.H., Fung J.J., Starzl T.E. (1991): Hepatology 13:619-626.
9. Lauchart W., Muller R., Pichlmayr R. (1987): Transplant. Proc., 19:4051-4053.
10. Samual D., Bismuth A., Mathieu D., Arulnaden J.L., Reynes M., Benhamou J.P., Brechat C., Bismuth H. (1991): Lancet, 337:813-815.
11. Shah G., Demetris A.J., Gavaler J.S., Lewis J.H., Todo S., Starzl T.E., Van Thiel D.H. (1991): Gastroenterology, (in press).
12. Tzakis A.G., Arditi M., Whitington P.F., Yanaka K., Esquivel C., Andrews W.A., Makowka L., Malatack J., Freese D.K., Stock P.G., Asher N.L., Johnson F.L., Broelsch C.E., Starzl T.E. (1988): N. Engl. J. Med., 319:393-396.
13. Van Thiel D.H., Carr B.I., Yokoyama I., Iwatsuki S., Starzl T.E. (1991): In: Etiology, pathology and treatment of hepatocellular carcinoma in North America, edited by E. Tabor, A.M. DiBisceglie, R.H. Purcell, pp. 309-316. Gulf Publishing Co., Houston, Texas.

14. Sakr M.F., Zetti G.M., Hassanein T.I., Farghali H., Nalesnik M.A., Gavaler J.S., Starzl T.E., Van Thiel D.H. (1991): Hepatology, 13:947-951.
15. DiBisceglie A.M. (1989): Seminars in Liver Disease, 9:254-258.
16. Van Thiel D.H., Gavaler J.S. (1991): In: Medicine North America, edited by C. Clegg, pp. 1894-1900. CME Publishing Ltd., Ontario, Canada.
17. Yokoyama I., Todo S., Iwatsuki S., Starzl T.E. (1990): Hepatogastroenterology, 37:188-193.
18. Esquivel C.O., Van Thiel D.H., Demetris A., Bernardos A., Iwatsuki S., Markus B., Gordon R.D., Marsh J.W., Makowka L., Tzakis A.G., Todo S., Gavaler J.S., Starzl T.E. (1988): Gastroenterology, 94:1207-1216.
19. Marsh J.W., Iwatsuki S., Makowka L., Esquivel C.O., Gordon R.D., Todo S., Tzakis A., Miller C., Van Thiel D.H., Starzl T.E. (1988): Ann. Surg., 207:21-25.
20. Higashi H., Yanaga K., Marsh J.W., Tzakis A., Kakizoe S., Starzl T.E. (1990): Hepatology, 11:477-480.

PRACTICAL USES OF OKT3

C.O. Esquivel, P. Nakazato, W. Concepcion, J.L. Szpakowski, C. Gettys, and J. Lim

INTRODUCTION

OKT3, a monoclonal antibody against the CD_3 cell population, was introduced to hepatic transplantation in the mid-1980s for the treatment of steroid resistant rejection (1-3). For didactic purposes, the indications for OKT3 therapy may be divided into three broad categories: 1) as a rescue therapy for steroid resistant rejection; 2) as prophylactic (induction) therapy; and, 3) as the initial therapy of rejection with the goal of eliminating high doses of steroids during the period of convalescence. The results for the first two indications have been the subject of several publications (1-4) and will not be addressed in this manuscript. Instead, we will report our experience with the use of OKT3 for the initial treatment of rejection. In addition, our experience with the use of this monoclonal antibody in patients with postoperative renal failure, positive crossmatches or ABO incompatibility will also be reported.

Patients and Methods

We performed a retrospective analysis of the medical records of 193 patients who underwent 214 liver transplants between March 25, 1988 and April 3, 1991. There were 127 adults (> 18 years of age) and 66 children (< 18 years of age). For the purpose of this analysis, 3 patients who died within 3 days of OLT were excluded.

The immunosuppression for induction consisted of cyclosporine, methylprednisolone at a dose of 0.3 mg/kg/d i.v. (defined as low dose steroids); and Minnesota antilymphocyte globulin, until an adequate therapeutic level of cyclosporine was obtained (5). In the presence of rejection, the patients were treated with a 10-14 day course of OKT3. In mild rejection or in dubious conditions, the patients received a single pulse of hydrocortisone 15 mg/kg/i.v., and a biopsy was performed. If, indeed, the diagnosis was rejection,

D. Galmarini et al. (eds.), Drugs and the Liver: High Risk Patients and Transplantation, 143–148.

the patients were given OKT3 treatment. OKT3 resistant rejection was treated with a steroid recycle for five days as reported elsewhere (6). In patients with positive crossmatches or renal failure or in those receiving organs across the ABO group, OKT3 was used for induction therapy.

RESULTS

Patient and Graft Survival

The overall patient and graft actuarial survival was 85% and 75%, respectively, at three years. Ninety-four patients received no OKT3 (Group I), because they had mild or no rejection at all. Ninety-five patients received OKT3; 66 for rejection (Group II), and 29 for induction therapy (Group III). A comparison of Group I vs. Groups II and III combined showed a patient survival of 90% and 80%, respectively, and the difference did not reach statistical significance. The corresponding graft survival was 80% and 75% for Group I vs. Groups II plus III, respectively (Fig. 1).

The comparison of Groups I and II combined vs. Group III yielded a patient survival of 90% and 75%, respectively, and there was a difference in graft survival as well (Fig. 2).

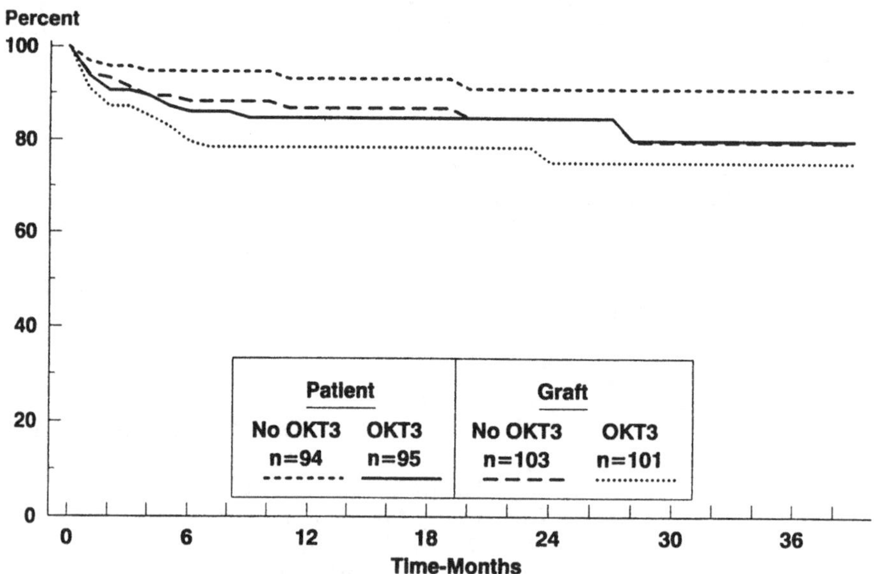

Fig 1. Comparison of patient and graft survival curves of liver transplant recipients receiving no OKT3 (Group I) vs those receiving OKT3(Groups II & III). The difference was not statistically significant ($p > 0.05$).

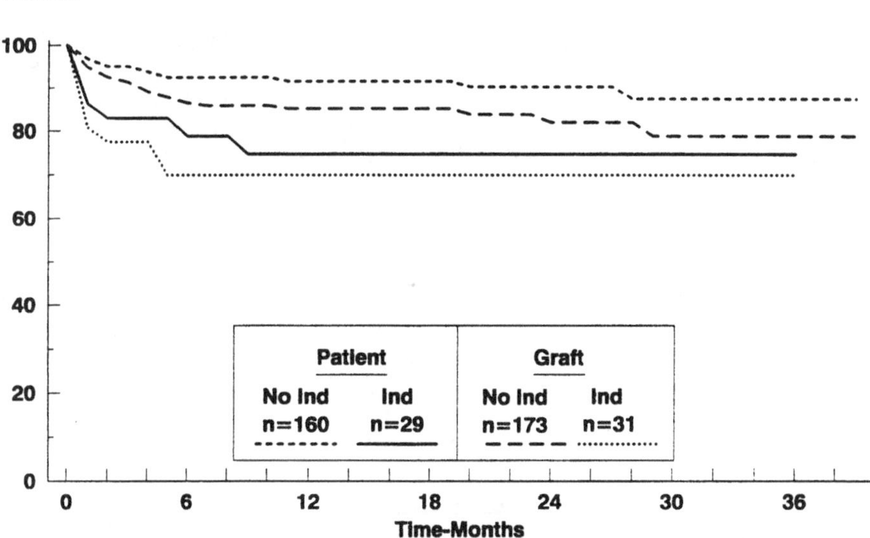

Fig 2. Comparison of patient and graft survival curves of liver transplant recipients receiving OKT3 for induction therapy (Group III) vs no OKT3 (Group 1 & Group II). The difference was significant in patient (p=0.0118) and graft survival (p=0.034) indicating that patients in Group III fall into a high risk category.

Retransplantation

The overall rate for retransplantation was 10%. For Group I the rate was 6%, Group II , 13%; and, Group III, 6%. The leading cause of graft loss was from extrahepatic causes (i.e. intraoperative death, myocardial infarction, MOSF due to sepsis, etc.). This was followed by primary graft nonfunction (19%), rejection (18%), and technical mishaps (13%). Further analysis showed that more grafts were lost due to rejection in Group II than were lost in Groups I and III (Table 1).

TABLE 1. Causes of Graft Loss n=47

	Rej	Tech	PNF	RecDx	Ex Hep
No OKT3	1	4	6	3	11
OKT3 Rejection	5	1	0	1	6
OKT3 Induction	1	1	3	2	2

Rej = rejection; Tech = technical complications; PNF = primary graft non-function; Rec Dx = recurrent disease; Ex Hep = extrahepatic causes.

Rejection

Seventy-seven percent of patients in Group II had at least one episode of rejection compared to 65% of the patients who received OKT3 for induction (Group III). In the entire series, only 23% of patients required high dose steroids, and most of them belonged to Group II.

Infection

The incidence and type of infections are reported in Table 2 and 3. Patients in Group I had a lower incidence of bacterial infections than Groups II or III. The incidence of viral and fungal infections was similar among the three groups (Table 3). Adults and children had a similar incidence of infections.

TABLE 2. Incidence of Infection

	Number	Percent	Episodes/ Patients
No OKT3	50/94	53%	0.9
OKT3-Rejection	51/66	77%	1.7
OKT3-Induction	24/29	83%	1.7

Lymphoproliferative Disorder (LPD)

In the entire series there were 8 cases (6%) of LPD, and all belonged to Group II. Seven of these patients were adults; four out of the 8 patients died (Table 4).

TABLE 3. Type of Infection

	Bacterial N (%)	Viral N (%)	Fungal N (%)
No OKT3	33 (35%)	24 (26%)	8 (9%)
OKT3-Rejection	40 (61%)	25 (38%)	11 (17%)
OKT3-Induction	19 (66%)	9 (31%)	6 (21%)
Overall	92 (49%)	58 (31%)	25 (13%)

DISCUSSION

As induction therapy, OKT3 was used only in patients who received ABO incompatible livers, in the presence of positive crossmatches, or in patients with postoperative renal failure in order to spare the use of CyA until the renal function recovered. Considering that this was a high-risk group of patients, our results showed that the patient and graft survival was satisfactory.

The most serious complication of OKT3 was an increased incidence of LPD in patients requiring OKT3 treatment for rejection and a similar observation was reported in heart transplant recipients (7). However, OKT3 may not be the only factor responsible for this increase since patients with frequent episodes of rejection usually receive more intense immunosuppression over all. Unlike previous reports, LPD affected mostly adult patients in our series (8). We do not have an explanation for this particular observation, but it is possible that adult patients require more intense immunosuppression than pediatric patients. Four of our patients who presented with mild hepatic dysfunction as the initial manifestation of LPD recovered well by reducing the dose of immunosuppression.

TABLE 4. Clinical Features of LPD

	Time to LPD (months)	Clinical Features	Outcome
1	1	Diffuse	Dead
2	1	Hepatitis	Alive (4 mos)
3	1	Hepatitis	Alive (4 mos)
4	3	Diffuse	Dead
5	2	Hepatitis	Alive (21mos)
6	12	Diffuse	Dead
7	2	Hepatitis	Alive (18 mos)
8	1	Diffuse	Dead

The goal of administering OKT3 as the initial therapy for rejection is to avoid high doses of steroids during the convalescence period. Steroids are well-known to impair wound healing and to predispose the patient to infections (9). Although our rate of infection is still significant, we feel that the number of fatal infections has decreased considerably, resulting in better patient and graft survival. Furthermore, a decrease in the rate of retransplantation was noted in patients who received OKT3 because of the decrease in the incidence of intractable rejection (2,3).

In conclusion, OKT3 therapy has become a practical and powerful tool in the immunosuppression of many liver transplant recipients.

REFERENCES

1. Starzl TE, Fung JJ. Orthoclone OKT3 intreatment of allografts rejected under cyclosporine-steroid therapy. Transplant Proc 18:937,1986.
2. Esquivel CO, Fung JJ, Markus B, et al. OKT3 in the reversal of acute hepatic allograft rejection. Transplant Proc 19:2443,1987.
3. Markus BH, Fung JJ, Gordon RD, et al. Effect of OKT3 on survival and rate of retransplantation. Transplant Proc 19:61,1987.
4. McDiarmid SV, Busuttil RW, Levy P, et al: The long-term outcome of OKT3 compared with cyclosporine prophylaxis after liver transplantation. Transplantation 52:01-97,1991.
5. Szpakowski J-L, Cox K, Nakazato P, et al. Experiences with the first 100 liver transplants at the Pacific Transplant Institute in San Francisco. Western J Med In Press.
6. Starzl TE, Iwatsuki S, Van Thiel DH: Evolution of liver transplantation. Hepatology 2:614-636,1982.
7. Swinnen LJ, Costanzo-Nordin MR, Fisher SG, et al: Increased incidence of lymphoproliferative disorder after immunosuppression with the monoclonal antibody OKT3 in cardiac transplant recipients. N Engl J Med 323:1723-28, 1990.
8. Nalesnik MA, Makowka L, Starzl TE: The diagnosis and treatment of posttransplant lymphoproliferative disorders. Curr Prob Surg 25:371-372,1988.
9. Gorensek MJ, Stewart RW, Keys TF: Decreased infections in cardiac transplant recipients on cyclosporine with reduced corticosteroid use. Clev J Med 56:690-5,1989.

HISTOPATOLOGY OF ACUTE LIVER REJECTION (ALR) IN OKT3 TREATED PATIENTS.

B.Gridelli, F.Donato, M.Colledan, G.Rossi, E.Melada, L.Caccamo, A.Lucianetti, L.P.Bonara, A.Colombo, M.Doglia, L.R.Fassati, D.Galmarini.

Over 70% of the patients that have received a liver allograft experience at least one episode of acute rejection from as early as 5 days after transplantation to months later. Most episodes of acute rejection however occur about 10 days after grafting when the patients'organ system is still recovering from a major surgical trauma. Accurate diagnosis and optimal treatment are major objectives in the postoperative treatment of liver transplant patients.

The classical histopathological signs of ALR are: 1) Mixed lymphocytic and granulocytic cellular infiltration of the portal tracts (Fig.1) and, incostantly, around the central

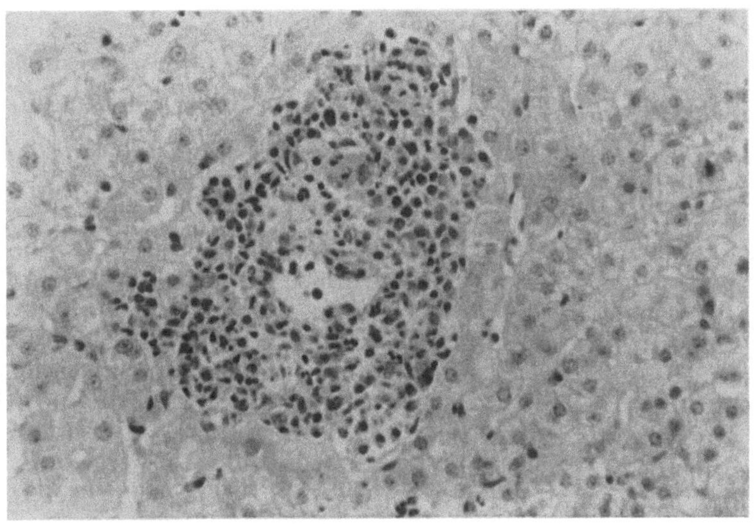

Fig.1: Portal tract of a needle liver biopsy taken eight days after OLTX (H & E, x 250).

D. Galmarini et al. (eds.), Drugs and the Liver: High Risk Patients and Transplantation, 149–154.

veins 2) Accumulation of lymphocytes on the endothelium and the walls of the portal and central veins 3) Bile duct damage (1). Other changes that are often present, but nonspecific, include bile stasis in centrilobular hepatocytes, bile thrombi in centrilobular bile canaliculi, ballooning of hepatocytes and small areas of mainly centrilobular necrosis. Arteritis, balloning and bile duct loss have been associated to episodes of acute rejection resistant to therapy (2).

Many of the histologic pictures found in acute rejection can be caused by other insults to the liver graft. Ischemic damage, viral infections and sepsis are conditions that can mimick, or coexist with acute rejection and that should be correctly diagnosed in order to plan the best therapeutic strategy.

More than 50% of the episodes of acute rejection respond to treatment with steroids. OKT3 has proven to be effective in the treatment of as many as 90% of steroid resistant rejections and as first line therapy of liver rejection (3,4). OKT3 exerts its effect on graft infiltrating and circulating CD3 lymphocytes providing at the same time powerful antirejection action and generalized immunosuppression that can favor the occurence of severe infections.

The study of liver biopsies is of paramount importance in deciding about the use of OKT3 in presence of liver graft disfunction and to monitor the effects of OKT3 therapy.

The objective of this study has been to verify wether any histologic feature of graft disfunction, before and after OKT3 therapy, had any prognostic value.

Patients and Methods

The records of 30 patients that underwent orthotopic liver transplantation at our institution and received OKT3 for the first time to treat an episode of ALR were reviewed. OKT3 was administered at a daily dose of 5 mg for adults and 2,5 mg for children. CD3 lymphocytes count was monitored during the OKT3 course and if CD3 percentage exceeded 10% the drug dose was doubled, if it exceeded 30% OKT3 was stopped because of inefficacy. The end transplant, pre- and post-OKT3 biopsies of these 30 patients were retrospectively reviewed and 26 histopathological signs of liver disfunction analyzed and graded for severity and/or distribution (3). Also white blood cell count (WBC), GOT, GGT and total bilirubin were computed. For the analysis of the numerical (hematology and biochemistry) and categorical (histology) data, the repeated measures analysis of the variance was performed. The differences of the considered parameters between surviving (S) and dying (D) patients were calculated using GLM and CATMOD procedures of the SAS statistics software (5). For each parameter also the interaction between time and mortality was considered. When present it was called positive time effect on mortality (PTEM). Student's test was used to analyze the differences in the duration of OKT3 therapy between S and D patients.

Results

The age of the patients ranged from 2 to 57 years (mean 32.3±15.2 SD) and the mean duration of OKT3 therapy was 13 days (± 3.6 SD). 23 patients are alive with a mean follow-up of 728 days (± 421 SD), while 7 patients died from 27 to 399 days aftert OLTX. In 4 patients death causes were mainly infective (CMV, aspergillus, EBV, bacterial sepsis) in 3 patients death was caused by rejection with or without infection.

In analyzing the differences between S and D patients a statistically significant difference in the duration of OKT3 treatment was evident, with D patients having had longer OKT3 courses (15.2±2.8 SD versus 12.9±2.3 SD days; p = 0.03). Statistically significant differences were also present in the liver function tests data. D patients had higher bilirubin levels before (p= 0.000) and after OKT3 (p= 0.029) when they also exhibited higher GGT levels (p=0.049). At the study of end-transplant liver biopsies no statistically significant differences were noted between D and S patients. D patients however had more bile duct damage in the biopsy performed before starting the OKT3 therapy for acute rejection (p=0.0016). No other histological parameter at this stage identified patients with poor prognosis.

The liver biopsies that were performed at the end of the OKT3 therapy were retrospectively more informative. D patients still had more severe bile duct epithelial damage (p= 0.0042); the statistical analysis also showed that the evolution of bile duct damage was different in D and S patients and that this evolution significantly influenced the final outcome of D patients (PTEM p=0.0182). The endothelialitis that was similarly present in D and S patients before OKT3, in S patients ameliorated with the treatment whereas in

D patients it remained unchanged (PTEM p = 0.0179). After OKT3, in D patients cholestasis, mainly centrilobular (Fig.2),was another tipical finding (p= 0.0026). This aspect suggested that a multifactorial liver graft damage was taking place since cholestasis is known to be caused also by ischemia and sepsis.

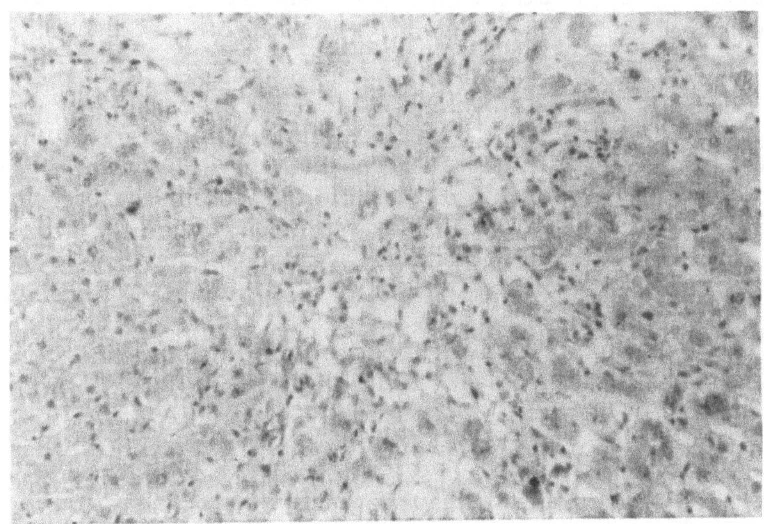

Fig.2. Needle liver biopsy at the end of a 14 day OKT3 course showing centrilobular cholestasis and ballooning of the hepatocytes (H & E x 250).

Discussion

The histological analysis of liver grafts has provided invaluable information on the causes of post-transplantation liver disfunction and also allowed the characterization and grading of rejection episodes. Serial liver biopsy studies are used to direct immunosuppression and to make previsions on the final outcome of ALR (2,6). We have tried to identify histological aspects whose evolution over a rather short period of time (duration of OKT3 therapy) could have a prognostic value for survival.

The results of our study indicate that patients that died had more severe episodes of rejection at the beginning of the OKT3 therapy as suggested both by biochemical and histological data. Even if there is no significant difference in the postoperative day of OKT3 course start between D and S patients, a delay in diagnosis might have played a role. The more severe biochemical data and histological pictures of these patients prompted more prolonged OKT3 courses that appear to have been ineffective in reversing the acute rejection episodes and probably had a major role in causing lethal infections.

Histologically the greater severity of ALR in D patients was expressed by the more intense and diffuse bile duct damage that was not reversed by therapy. The vascular endothelium of the portal and centrilobular veins is another important target of the immune attack of the graft. While at the beginning of the rejection episode endothelialitis was equally present in D and S patients only in the latter the trend during OKT3 course was toward a regression of the vascular lesions. In D patients the occurrence of an uncontrolled immunologically mediated impairment of graft vascular supply was also suggested by the centrilobular cholestasis that became more evident at the end of OKT3 treatment. On the basis of this experience it seems that graft disfunction should be precociusly and carefully investigated with liver biopsy to properly grade the severity of the eventual rejection episode. This policy should allow to start of proper antirejection therapy before the lesions become too severe.

The data of this study need further validation with analysis of more patients but we suggest that it is possible to identify histological pictures whose evolution during a fairly short period of time can have a prognostic value for survival.

References

1) Demetris J.A., Lasky A., Van Thierl D.H., Starzl T.E., Dekker A.(1984): Am. J. Path., 118: 151-161.

2) Snover D.C., Freese D.K., Sharp H.L., Bloomer J.R., Najariean J.S., Asdcher N.L.(1987): Am. J. Surg. Pathol., 1987, 11:1-10.

3) Busuttil R.W. (1989): Transplant Proc., 21: 19-23.

4) Muhlbacker F., Staininger R., Langle F., Hamilton G., Sautner T., Gnant M., Gotzinger P., Piza F., Popow T.: Transplant.Proc., 21: 25-30.

5) Catmod Procedure in: SAS Institute Inc. SAS/STAT[tm] User's Guide Release 6.03 Edition Cory, NC: SAS Institute Inc., 1988.

6) Williams J.W., Peter T.G., Vera S.G., Britt L.C., Van Voorst S.J., Haggit R.C.(1985): Transplantation, 39: 589-596.

SPIN-SPIN RELAXATION TIMES AS VIABILITY PARAMETER OF LIVER TRANSPLANTATION GRAFTS. INVESTIGATION ON A PIG MODEL

P.Holzmüller, E.Moser, R.Steininger , H.Reckendorfer , W.Feigl , M.Sperlich and H.Burgmann

INTRODUCTION

Primary graft non function is an unsolved problem in liver transplantation surgery since there is no possibility to determine organ viability and post transplant graft function before implantation. Previous investigations on a rat model showed highly significant correlations of proton nuclear magnetic resonance (NMR) spin-spin relaxation times (T_2) of livers, stored in different protecting solutions, and viability parameters (1 - 3), encouraging us to investigate our simple, rapid and cheap method on an other species and also in men.

MATERIAL AND METHODS

In this test series ortotopic liver transplantation was performed on pigs and graft NMR relaxation times were assessed. Two liver protective solutions, the University of Wisconsin- (UW)- and Bretschneider´s- HTK solution, were compared to investigate different effects of storage. Two storage times were investigated : 90 minutes, the shortest possible delay between organ harvesting and implantation, and 24 hours storage, a period where no positive outcome was expected. Storage temperature was 4°C. The number of animals used was as follows : UW short time n = 4, UW long time n = 5, HTK short time n = 3, HTK long time n = 5.

Liver biopsies were collected immediately after opening of the abdomen and prior to implantation.

T_2 was determined 30 minutes after biopsy excision using a low resolution ^{1}H-NMR spectrometer (minispec pc120, 0.47T Bruker, Karlsruhe, FRG) and applying a CPMG pulse sequence (T_E = 2 ms, N = 100, T_R = 3.0 s, 9 averages). Measurement

D. Galmarini et al. (eds.), Drugs and the Liver: High Risk Patients and Transplantation, 155–158.

temperature was 37°C. A monoexponential model was fitted for quantitative data analysis.

Overall hepatic tissue water content was estimated gravimetrically and is given in percent wet weight.

The evaluation of tissue damage was performed by light microscopy.

High energy phosphate levels were assessed by HPLC and energy charge was calculated according to Atkinson.

$$\text{energy charge} = \frac{\text{ATP} + 0.5\ \text{ADP}}{\text{AMP} + \text{ADP} + \text{ATP}}$$

Statistical data treatment : mean data values ± one sample standard deviation are given. Good and poor liver protection was compared using Mann-Whitney U test. Differences were considered of significance with $p < 0.05$.

RESULTS

90 minutes of storage left the organs almost unaltered whereas 24 hours of cold storage resulted in liver damage independent of the protective solution used, as was confirmed histologically. After 24 hours storage considerable sinusoidal dilatation, pyknosis of sinusoidal endothelial cells and intracellular vacuolization was evident.

Due to the large data scatter obtained from normal pig liver ($T_2 = 46.5 \pm 4.1$ ms, water content = 74.5 ± 1.3 %, energy charge = 0.60 ± 0.15) only the use of Δ-values was appropriate.

Significant differences between good and poor UW protection occurred for ΔT_2, ΔATP and Δenergy charge (fig. 1 and 2). No significant differences were found for Δwater content despite a clear trend to decrease with storage time was evident (fig. 3).

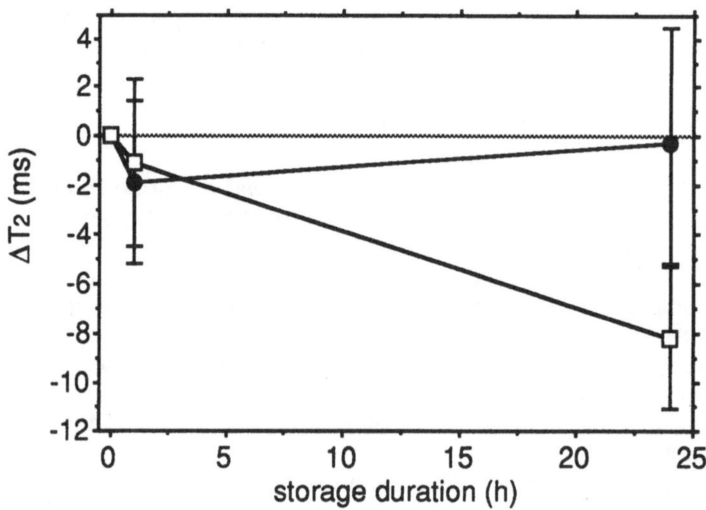

FIG. 1 : ΔT_2 in milliseconds versus storage duration in hours. Organs protected in HTK (●)- or UW (□) solution.

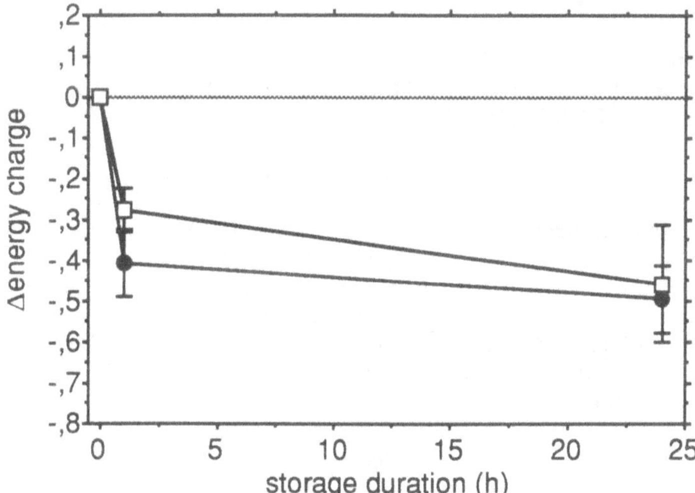

FIG. 2 : Δenergy charge versus storage duration in hours. Organs protected in HTK (●)- or UW (□) solution.

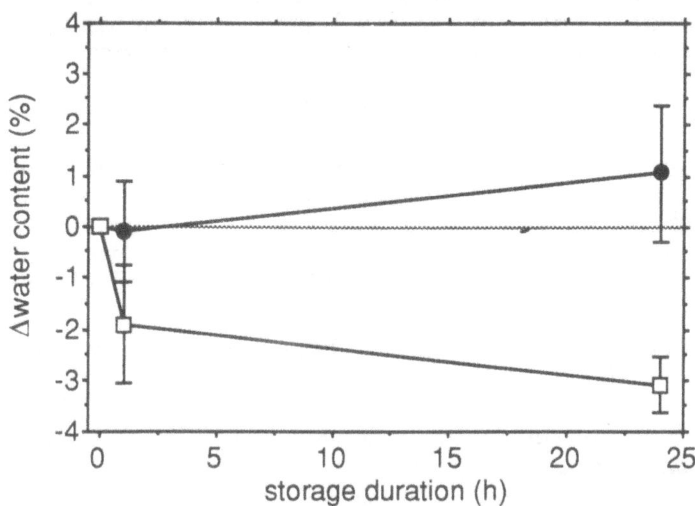

FIG. 3 : Δwater content in percent versus storage duration in hours. Organs protected in HTK (●)- or UW (□) solution.

However, no significant differences were detected for any parameter between good and poor HTK storage (figs. 1 - 3).

Highly significant correlations between ΔT_2 and Δwater content (HTK : $R = 0.80$, $p < 0.001$; UW : $R = 0.85$, $p < 0.001$) for both storage solutions were detected.

Also highly significant correlations between ΔT_2, ΔATP and Δenergy charge for UW (ΔT_2/ΔATP : $R = 0.75$, $p < 0.005$; ΔT_2/Δenergy charge : $R = 0.73$, $p < 0.005$)

occurred.

Highly significant correlations were found between Δwater content, ΔATP and Δenergy charge for UW (Δwater content/ΔATP : $R = 0.84$, $p < 0.001$; Δwater content/ Δenergy charge : $R = 0.89$, $p < 0,001$).

CONCLUSIONS

Good and poor protection of donor livers stored in UW solution is reflected by T_2 relaxation times, showing a highly significant correlation with tissue water content and high energy phosphate levels. Water content is assumed to be a valuable parameter of liver viability as it reflects tissue edema and cell integrity. The major disadvantage of water content estimation for viability testing is the amount of time necessary. Our method solves this problem and provides accurate data 30 minutes after biopsy excision.

However, it was not possible to assess organ quality of HTK protected pig liver. HTK seems to provide homeostasis of cellular water content longer than it protects tissue viability in this species. This leads to the conclusion that one has to be careful in drawing general conclusions from our results. Each storage solution has to be investigated separately whether viability detection using NMR relaxometry is possible or not. Fortunately this method seems to work with UW solution which is the gold standard of liver protective solutions today.

Thus, it should be possible to establish a quick viability testing protocol, based on our method and complementary tests, for UW protected human transplantation liver.

Further investigations on human liver biopsies are in progress.

ACKNOWLEDGEMENTS

Work supported by the Austrian Fonds zur Förderung der wissenschaftlichen Forschung, under grant P7017 Med, and by the Jubiläumsfonds der österreichischen Nationalbank, under grant 3687.

REFERENCES

1. Holzmüller P., Reckendorfer H., Burgmann H. and Moser E. (1990): *Magn.Res.Med.*, 16: 173-178.

2. Moser E., Holzmüller P., Reckendorfer H. and Burgmann H. (1991): *Transplantation*, in press

3. Burgmann H., Reckendorfer H., Holzmüller P., Moser E., Spieckermann P.G. (1990): *Transplant.Proc.*, 23: 1974.

URINARY 6-ß HYDROXYCORTISOL AS A PREDICTOR OF CYCLOSPORINE BLOOD LEVELS

A. LEMOINE , T. BIENVENU , D. AZOULAY , L. KIFFEL , M. JOHANN , D. SAMUEL and H. BISMUTH

The cytochrome P-450 IIIA, a major constitutive isoenzyme of human liver drug-metabolizing enzymes, is responsible for the metabolism of cyclosporine (CSA) (1,2,3). The catalytic activity of this isoenzyme varies up to twenty-fold between patients and could explain the wide individual variability in plasma levels upon administration of equal doses (2). This may have implications for its benefits and risks (e.g. neurotoxicity and renal failure) (4). In general, renal and neurological toxicities of CSA are associated with high levels of drug in blood. However, CSA can induce renal and neurological dysfunctions in some patients while blood levels of parent drug are not elevated (5, 6).

Two different methods are currently available to evaluate the hepatic level of cytochrome P-450 IIIA :

- the direct immunoquantification in liver by western blotting (3),
- [^{13}C or ^{14}C]-erythromycin breath test (3), an indirect method.

However, these methods are very complex, expensive, and difficult to realize routinely.

As P-450 IIIA catalyzes endogenous cortisol into 6ß-hydroxycortisol, a metabolite completely eliminated in urines (7), the ability of patients to produce 6ß-hydroxycortisol might be useful in predicting an appropriate initial dosing regimen for CSA.

MATERIALS

- Liver biopsies from 13 liver allografts (10 males and 3 females, median age: 47, extremes: 24-61) were collected during transplantation in "Service du Pr Bismuth - Hôpital Paul Brousse - Villejuif - France".
- All patients received 1 mg/kg CSA daily, from day 1 to day 3 after transplantation.
- Urine samples were collected one day after transplantation.
- CSA monitoring was performed daily.

D. Galmarini et al. (eds.), Drugs and the Liver: High Risk Patients and Transplantation, 159–163.

METHODS

- Cytochrome P-450 isozymes (P-450 IA, IIC, IID, IIIA) were quantified by western blotting. Briefly 50 μg homogenate proteins were separated by sodium dodecyl sulfate-polyacrylamide gel electrophoresis (9%) and transferred onto nitrocellulose. Cytochrome P-450 was detected by the antiperoxidase technique. The stained bands were quantified by reflecting scanning and subsequent integration using computer design program IMSTAR. Results were expressed as a relative concentration of the tested cytochrome P-450 in each liver biopsy compared to the intensity of 5μg of the corresponding cytochrome P-450 antigen. We used monoclonal antibody P-450-IIIA and polyclonal antibodies raised against cytochrome P-450 IA, IIC, and IID (supplied by Pr Ph. Beaune and Dr. Kiffel, Hôpital Necker, Paris).
- CSA blood levels were measured by radioimmunoassay in whole blood using polyclonal antibody. Results were expressed as the mean of CSA blood levels of the first three days after transplantation.
- 6ß-hydroxycortisol was quantified by HPLC in urine samples according to the technique described by Ged et al. (7).

RESULTS

- Immunoblot analysis (figure 1A) showed a wide variability (5 fold) in relative hepatic concentration of cytochrome P-450 IIIA between 13 samples (extremes: 11-51).

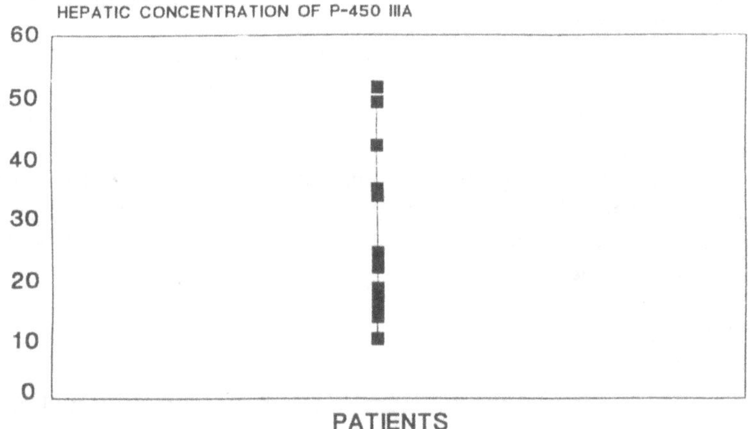

FIG.1A, variability in relative concentration of cytochrome P-450 IIIA determined by western blotting between 13 patients.

Figure 1B showed a large individual variability (8 fold) in CSA blood levels.

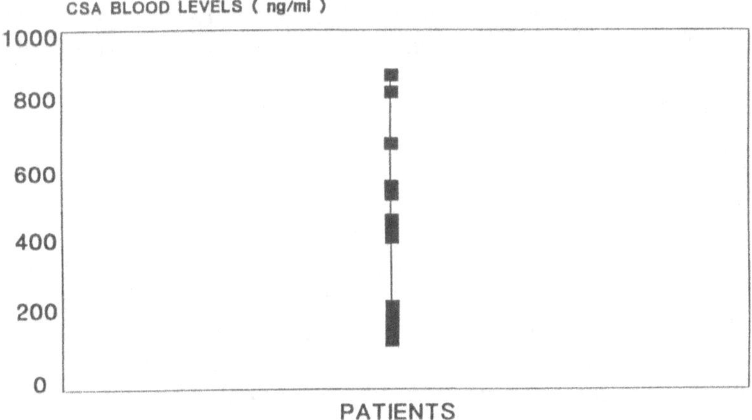

FIG. 1B, variability in CSA blood levels between 13 patients.

- The comparison of variability of the different hepatic cytochromes P-450 content showed no correlation between CSA and cytochromes P-450 IA, IIC, IID, but two groups have been distinguished for cytochrome P-450 IIIA content (figure 2):

Group 1 with low hepatic cytochrome P-450 IIIA content (<20, n=5) and high CSA blood levels (675 ± 173 ng/ml),

Group 2 with high hepatic cytochrome P-450 IIIA content (>20, n=8) and low CSA blood levels (269 ± 173 ng/ml).

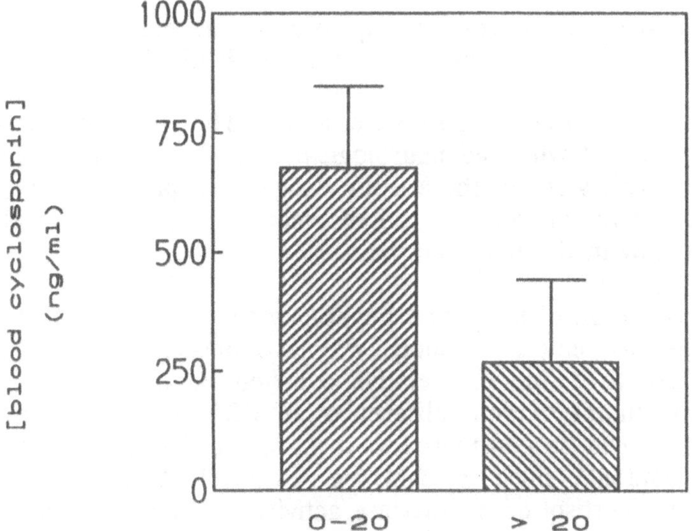

FIG. 2, comparison of variability of CSA blood levels and cytochrome P-450 IIIA content.

- Urinary 6ß-hydroxycortisol concentration, measured in 6 patients, showed a trend to linear correlation with hepatic cytochrome P-450 IIIA content ($r=0.689$). No correlation has been obtained between cytochrome P-450 IA, IIC, IID and CSA blood levels or urinary 6ß-hydroxycortisol.

DISCUSSION

This *in vivo* study has confirmed that the variations of CSA blood levels in treated patients were related to the immunochemically detected signal of hepatic cytochrome P-450 IIIA content.
Involvement of a single cytochrome P-450, i.e. cytochrome P-450 IIIA, in the formation of CSA metabolism in liver has been principally studied in the rabbit (1). Using microsomes of 15 human livers, Kronbach et al. (2), have shown the dose dependent and almost complete inhibition of all three main metabolites (two monohydroxylated M1 and M17, and the demethylated M21 metabolites) by antibodies raised against cytochrome P-450 IIIA.
In vivo, no linear correlation has been obtained between CSA blood levels and hepatic cytochrome P-450 IIIA content, presumably due to the results of the different techniques used to measure activity and proteins. Radioimmunoassay has been used for CSA blood levels determination with a polyclonal antibody that cross-reacts with the metabolites of CSA and therefore is unable to differentiate between the parent compound and its metabolites (8).
However, we have distinguished two groups of patients: one group with low P-450 IIIA concentration and high CSA blood levels and the second group with high hepatic P-450 IIIA concentration and low CSA blood levels.
Since P-450 IIIA may detoxify or help to eliminate metabolites generated by other enzymes, deficiency in cytochrome P-450 IIIA activity would therefore result in accumulation of the parent drug or accumulation of toxic metabolites as described Lucey et al. (3). They have observed a liver transplant recipient who had neurological and renal failure whereas his CSA blood levels were in therapeutic range. The patient died during a second transplantation and the microsomal content of P-450 IIIA was found to be low in the first transplant.

Because evaluation of individual hepatic cytochrome P-450 IIIA content was not easy to realize routinely, we have measured the urinary 6ß-hydroxycortisol to define the relative contribution of cytochrome P-450 heterogeneity in interpatient differences in CSA tolerance. Indeed, 6ß-hydroxycortisol can be considered as a marker of hepatic cytochrome P-450 IIIA content, since cytochrome P-450 IIIA is predominantly responsible for cortisol 6ß-hydroxylase activity in human liver microsomes and urinary 6ß-hydroxycortisol levels correlated with hepatic P-450 IIIA specific content (7).

The urinary metabolite of an endogenous compound measurement is a non invasive technique in comparison to [^{13}C]erythromycin breath test, previously used as a marker of hepatic cytochrome P-450 IIIA content (3). The correlation obtained between urinary 6ß-hydroxycortisol and cytochrome P-450 IIIA content was low ($r=0.689$) because of the small number of points (6 patients). However, a previous study (7) in a larger population ($n=22$) has shown a close correlation ($r= 0.830$; $p<0.001$).

These results are currently undergoing in a larger population to confirm if the non invasive urinary 6ß-hydroxycortisol assay will provide useful information to adjust the initial and individual dose of CSA to ensure efficacy/security of the therapeutic treatment of this immunosuppressive agent.

Urinary 6ß-hydroxycortisol could also be useful in preventing interactions on CSA blood levels of drugs such as phenytoin, barbiturates, rifampicine, ketoconazole, methylprednisolone, erythromycin, dilthiazem, nicardipine, verapamil, and sulfamethazine that complicate CSA therapy (9, 10, 11, 12).

Taking together these results, an alternative therapeutic approach, in case of low urinary 6ß-hydroxycortisol concentration, could consist in: 1) decreasing the initial dose per kg of CSA or 2) increasing the cytochrome P-450 IIIA activity by xenobiotics such as rifampicine that is known to induce this cytochrome P-450 (3).

BIBLIOGRAPHY

1. Bertault-pères P., Bonfils C., Fabre G., Just S., Cano J.P., and Maurel P. (1897):Drug Metab. Dispos., 15: 391-397.
2. Kronbach T., Fischer V. and Meyer U.A. (1988): Clin. Pharmacol. Ther., 43: 630-635.
3. Lucey M.R., Kolars J.C., Merion R.M., Campbell D.A., Aldrich M., and Watkins P.B. (1990): Lancet, 35: 11-15.
4. Ptachinski R.J., Venkataramanan R., and Burckart G.J. (1986), Clin. Pharmacokin., 11: 107-132.
5. Kahan B.D. and Grevel J. (1988): Transplantation, 46: 631-644.
6. De Groen P.C., Aksanut A.J., Rakela J., Forbes G.S. and Krom R.A.F. (1987): N. Engl. J. Med., 317: 861-866.
7. Ged C., Rouillon J.M., Pichard L., Combalbert J., Bressot N., Michel H., Beaune P. and Maurel P. (1989): Br. J. Clin. Pharmacol., 28: 373-387.
8. Donats P., Abish E., Homberger M., Trahar R. and Trapp M. (1981): Journal of immunoassay, 2: 19-32.
9. Drug interactions of cyclosporine (1986): Aust. J. Pharm., 67: 848-849.
10. Godin J.R.P., Sketris I.S. and Belitsky P. (1986): Drug Intell. Clin. Pharm., 20: 504-505.
11. Pochet J.M. and Pirson Y. (1986): Lancet, i:979.
12. Lindhom A. and Henricsson S. (1987): Lancet, i:1262-1263.

ELUCIDATION OF THE METABOLIC PATHWAYS OF CYCLOSPORINE IN VITRO BY HUMAN LIVER MICROSOMES

U. Christians, H.M. Schiebel, J. Bleck and K.-Fr. Sewing

INTRODUCTION

Interest has focused on the ciclosporin metabolism and on the biological activity of ciclosporin metabolites since several clinical cases and studies were reported, in which increased blood concentrations of ciclosporin metabolites were associated with neuro-and nephrotoxicity (1-5). Further assessment of the toxic potential of ciclosporin metabolites and the underlying mechanisms, requires a detailed understanding of the metabolic pathways of ciclosporin.

It was the aim of the present study:
1) to study further metabolism of ciclosporin metabolites from human bile, by the use of human liver microsomes, to isolate these new metabolites from the microsomal preparations and to elucidate their structures and
2) to extend the known ciclosporin metabolic pathways to include these new metabolites.

METHODS

Metabolism of ciclosporin by human liver microsomes

Human liver microsomes were isolated using standard centrifugation techniques as described before by Guengerich et al (6). Ciclosporin and its metabolites were dissolved in methanol and 8.3 nmol were added to 1 ml of the microsomal suspension (3 mg protein/ml). The reaction was started by adding 0.5 ml of an NADPH regenerating system based on isocitrate dehydrogenase. The reaction was stopped by adding 0.5 ml acetonitrile, the first step of the extraction procedure.

After stopping the reaction the samples were centrifuged (2500 g, 2 min) and the supernatant was sucked through the extraction columns, filled with C8-

D. Galmarini et al. (eds.), Drugs and the Liver: High Risk Patients and Transplantation, 165–170.

material. The samples were washed with methanol/water pH 3.0 (50/50, v/v) and hexane. Ciclosporin and its metabolites were eluted with dichloromethane. Dichloromethane was evaporated, the samples were reconstituted in the mobile phase and washed with hexane before injection into the HPLC.

HPLC

Water at pH 3.0 and acetonitrile were used as eluents. Ciclosporin and its metabolites were eluted by a concave gradient (time 0 min: 42% acetonitrile, time 20 min: 46%, time 35 min: 65%, and time 55 min: 73%). The oven temperature was 75 °C, the UV detector wavelength 205 nm. For HPLC two subsequently linked columns were used: a 250x4 mm and a 100x4mm column, filled with 3 μm, C8 material.

FAB-MS

Fractions containing the same metabolite were pooled and extracted from the mobile phase using dichloromethane. Dichloromethane was evaporated and the residues were dissolved in the FAB-MS matrix, a mixture of dithiothreitol/ dithioerythritol 5:1.

Investigations of the metabolic pathway

Isolated metabolites were metabolized by human liver microsomes. The resulting metabolites were isolated by HPLC and their structures were checked by FAB-MS. By repetitive further metabolism, isolation and structural identification it was possible to follow the metabolic pathways of individual metabolites.

RESULTS

Fourteen metabolites, whose structures have not yet been elucidated were isolated after metabolism of structurally identified ciclosporin metabolites, and the chemical structures for 5 of these metabolites were proposed:
(i) an N-demethylated, carboxylated derivative (AM1A4N),
(ii) a di-hydroxylated, N-demethylated derivative (AM14N9),
(iii) a hydroxylated and carboxylated derivative (AM1A9),
(iv) a di-hydroxylated, cyclized and N-demethylated derivative (AM1c4N9) and
(v) a cyclized and carboxylated derivative.
All metabolites isolated during this study are listed in table 1.

A proposed ciclosporin metabolic pathway comprises a total of twenty-nine metabolites and consisted of four main branches originating from metabolites AM1, AM9, AM1c and AM4N (Fig. 1-4). Metabolite AM1c-Glc, which is a glucuronylated metabolite, could not be produced in vitro and its position in the metabolic pathway was not identified.

TABLE 1: Ciclosporin metabolites produced by and isolated from human liver microsomes or isolated from human bile

The reference numbers in column 1 correspond to those in the upper left corner of the ciclosporin metabolites in figures 1-4. The nomenclature of the Hawk's Cay consensus conference (1990) is listed in column 2, the retention times in the analytical h.p.l.c. assay in column 3, the molecular ion in the negative FAB mass spectrum in column 4 and the metabolic changes of the molecule from that of ciclosporin in column 5. Abbreviations: R_t: retention time in the analytical h.p.l.c. assay as described in the method section, Cs: ciclosporin.

#	nomenclature	R_t [min]	$[M-H]^-$ m/z	metabolic changes
1	AM1	39.6	1217.4	Cs + O
2	AM11d	38.2	1233.4	Cs + 2 O
3	AM1c	41.2	1217.4	Cs + O + cyclization
4	AM19	27.7	1233.6	Cs + 2 O
5	AM1AL	42.4/42.7	1215.4	Cs + O - 2 H
6	-	39.0	1231.4	Cs + 2 O - 2 H
7	AM1A	37.5	1231.4	Cs + 2 O - 2 H
8	-	25.8	1247.4	Cs + 3 O - 2 H
9	AM1A4N	23.0	1217.4	Cs + 2 O - 2 H - CH_3
10	-	21.6	1263.4	Cs + 4 O - 2 H
11	AM9	40.6	1217.4	Cs + O
12	AM1A9	26.4	1247.4	Cs + 3 O - 2 H
13	AM14N9	21.2	1219.4	Cs + 2 O - CH_3
14	-	25.3	1249.4	Cs + 3 O
15	-	21.3	1265.4	Cs + 4 O
16	AM4N	43.6	1187.4	Cs - CH_3
17	AM4N9	33.7	1203.4	Cs + O - CH_3
18	AM49	30.2	1233.4	Cs + 2 O
19	AM69	35.0	1233.6	Cs + 2 O
20	AM1Ac	32.1	1231.6	Cs + 2 O - 2 H + cyclization
21	AM1c9	29.6	1233.4	Cs + 2 O + cyclization
22	AM1c-Glc	26.6	1393.4	Cs + O + cyclization + glucuronylation
23	AM1c4N9	21.0	1219.4	Cs + 2 O - CH_3 + cyclization
24	-	24.9	1249.4	Cs + 3 O + cyclization
25	-	34.6	1203.4	Cs + O - CH_3
26	AM14N	31.2	1203.4	Cs + O - CH_3
27	AM4N69	28.9	1219.4	Cs + 2 O - CH_3
28	-	29.9	1219.4	Cs + 2 O - CH_3
29	-	21.2	1235.4	Cs + 3 O - CH_3

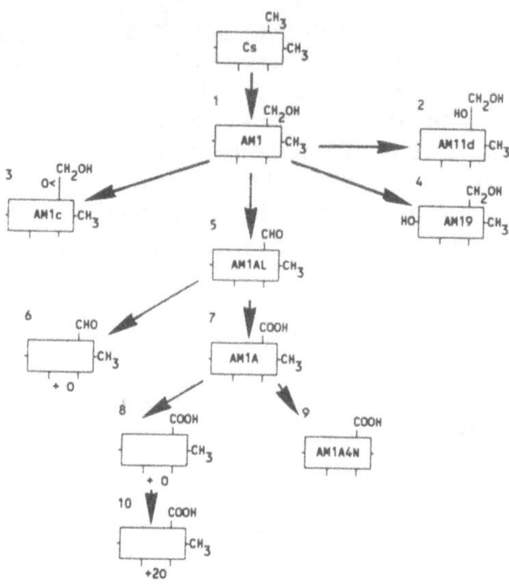

FIG. 1: Metabolic pathways of ciclosporin via AM1 as elucidated human microsomal metabolism. The reference numbers at the upper left corner of the metabolites refer to those of table 1.

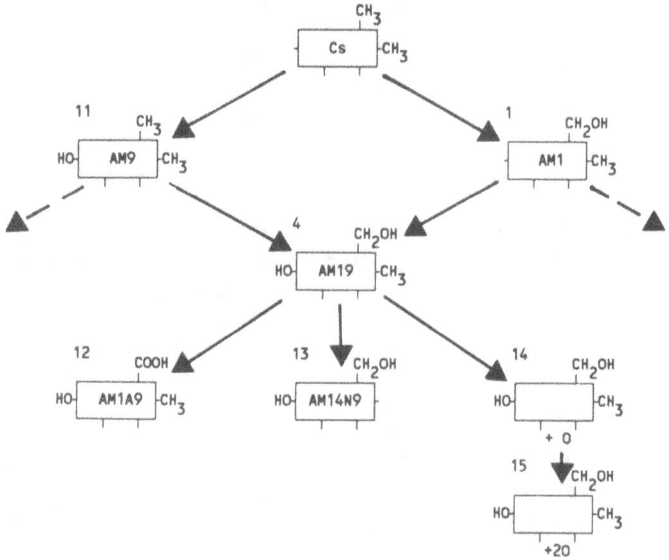

FIG. 2: Metabolic pathways of ciclosporin via AM19.

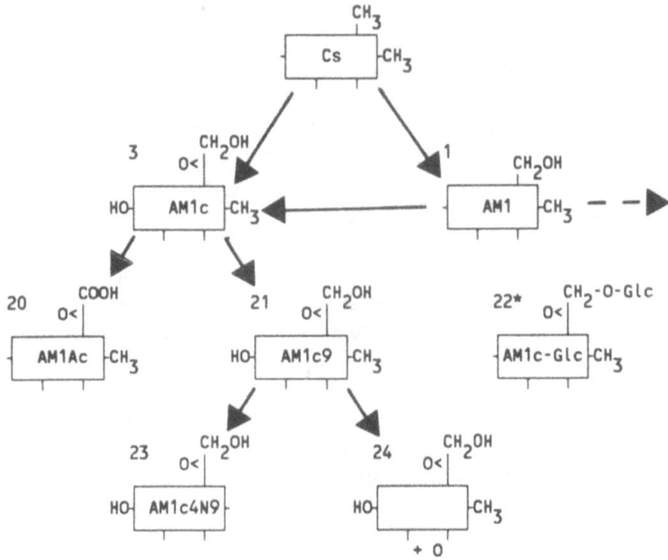

FIG. 3: Metabolic pathways via AM1c.
Metabolites, whose pathways could not be identified, are marked by *.

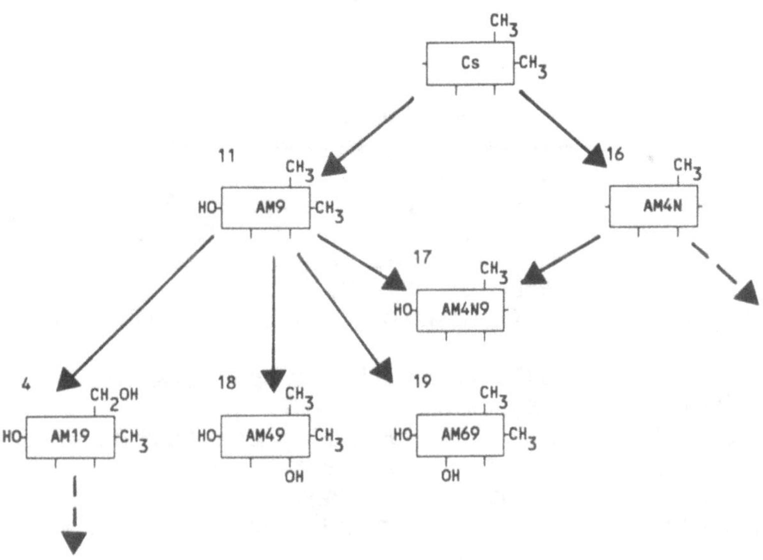

FIG. 4: Metabolic pathways of ciclosporin via AM9.

DISCUSSION

In the present study 14 metabolites, whose structures have not yet been defined, were formed by metabolism of isolated ciclosporin metabolites by microsomal preparations from human liver. The chemical structures of five of these metabolites could be derived from their mass spectra and the well defined structures of their parent compounds (table 1).

In the proposed metabolic pathways only the routes which could be confirmed by the in vivo experiments were displayed (fig. 1-4). The chemical structures of the metabolites imply that more cross-links between the metabolic pathway are possible than indicated by Wenger (7). It has to be taken into account that some short living metabolites were formed, so that their concentrations decreased below the detection limit before the assay was terminated. Thus some intermediate metabolites may not have been detected.

The metabolism of cyclized metabolites was of special interest, since there were only uncertain, indirect signs of cyclization of amino acid 1 in the mass spectra (8). Formation of a metabolite from a cyclized parent compound is likely to result in an also cyclized metabolite, so that these metabolites could clearly be identified. Metabolite AM1c can originate not only from AM1 but also directly from ciclosporin. This suggests the occurrence of a non-hydroxylated, cyclized ciclosporin derivative (AMc) as a precursor of AM1c. This hypothesis awaits confirmation.

The metabolism of purified and structurally well characterized metabolites by microsomes, subsequent isolation of the metabolites generated by HPLC and characterization by FAB-MS proved to be a valuable strategy to elucidate the metabolic pathway and to gain structural information about metabolites.

REFERENCES

1. Wonigeit K., Kohlhaw K., Winkler M., Schaefer O. and Pichlmayr R. (1990): Transplant. Proc. 22(3): 1305-1311.
2. Kohlhaw K., Wonigeit K., Schäfer O., Ringe B., Bunzendahl H. and Pichlmayr R. (1989): Transplant. Proc. 21: 2232-2233.
3. Kunzendorf U., Brockmüller J., Joachimsen F., Keller F., Waltz G. and Offermann G. (1988): Lancet 1: 1223.
4. Leunissen K., Baumann G., Bosmann R. and Van Hoof J.P. (1986): Lancet 2: 1398.
5. Lucey M.R., Kolars J.C., Merion R.M., Campbell D.A., Aldrich M. and Watkins P.B. (1990): Lancet 335: 11-15.
6. Guengerich F.P. (1982): In: Principles and methods of toxicology, edited by A.W. Hayes pp. 609-634. Raven Press, New York.
7. Wenger R.M. (1990): Transplant. Proc. 22(3): 1104-1108.
8. Wallemacq P.E., Lhoëst G., Latinne D. and de Bruyere M. (1989): Transplant. Proc. 21: 906-910.

ACKNOWLEDGEMENTS

The study was supported by DFG grant Pi48/11-4, project D5.

FINE-NEEDLE ASPIRATION BIOPSY AND HEPATOTOXICITY OF CYCLOSPORIN A IN ORTHOTOPIC LIVER TRANSPLANTATION

P. Palazzi, M. Parenti, R. Rivolta, A. Lucianetti , R. Romito , B. Gridelli .

INTRODUCTION

Fine-needle aspiration biopsy (FNAB) was originally developed for renal allografts (1) and then applied to liver transplantation in humans (2).

It represents a rapid and atraumatic method to diagnose and monitor the different causes of dysfunction after orthotopic liver transplantation. By this technique cellular infiltrates and parenchimal cell's morphology are analyzed.

Cyclosporin A (CSA) hepatotoxicity increases serum liver enzymes and bilirubin with an histological picture ranging from swelling of the hepatocytes and centrolobular fatty changes to centrolobular necrosis.

FNAB allows to characterize and differentiate CSA hepatotoxicity from the other causes of liver dysfunction (acute rejection, cholestasis, cholangitis, viral or bacterial infection, recurrence of the original disease) by the presence of a typical isometric vacuolization of the hepatocytes and the endothelial cells.

In this study we correlate parenchimal cell's morphology, CSA blood levels and the clinical outcome of the patients after drug reduction.

MATERIAL AND METHODS

We performed 85 liver FNABs in 28 patients 7,11 and 15 days after orthotopic liver transplantation (OLTX) or whenever an hepatic dysfunction occurred.

To compare the diagnosis 50 core biopsies were simultaneously performed.

D. Galmarini et al. (eds.), Drugs and the Liver: High Risk Patients and Transplantation, 171–176.

The technique to obtain and process FNAB was that described by Hayry et al. (1) for the kidney grafts.

The aspiration specimens of liver and blood were drown into a syringe containing Hepes buffered tissue culture medium. The material cytocentrifuged on microscope slides and stained with May-Grunwald Giemsa (MGG) were evaluated for:

Inflammatory infiltrate: this is determined by the increment method that emploies different correction factors to score the inflammatory cells involved in acute rejection (lymphoid blasts, plasma cells, monoblasts, macrophages, activated lymphocytes, monocytes, polymorphonuclear cells).

We obtained a total corrected increment (T.C.I.), parameter indicative of immunitary activation when > 3.5. A mild lymphoid activation with a few blasts cells and large granular lymphocytes (LGL) in both FNAB and blood specimens was seen during viral infections (3).

The presence of macrophages (> 1-2%) was considered suggestive for severe advanced and irreversible rejection or for intra or extraparenchimal collection.

Morphological changes of the epatocytes: the degenerative changes are usually scored from 1 to 4, indicating: 1= swelling, 2= swelling and vacuolization, 3= swelling, vacuolization and inclusions, 4= necrosis.

A typical isometric cytoplasmatic vacuolization of the hepatocytes is seen in CSA hepatotoxicity (fig.1); swelling, irregular vacuolization and/or bile droplets in hepatocytes are recordered during acute rejection;necrotic cells indicated severe tissue damage.

The specimens are considered representative if contained 7 or more than 7 hepatocytes for 100 nucleated cells. Specimens are also taken from patients with liver insufficiency and platelet count of 20.000/mm3.

The trough levels of CSA were measured on whole blood by RIA kit Sandoz utilizing a monoclonal aspecific antibody; the statistical analysis of these levels in the patients with cellular damage of CSA and in those without morphological changes of the hepatocytes was made by Student's t test.

No severe complication was observed after fine-needle aspiration biopsy.

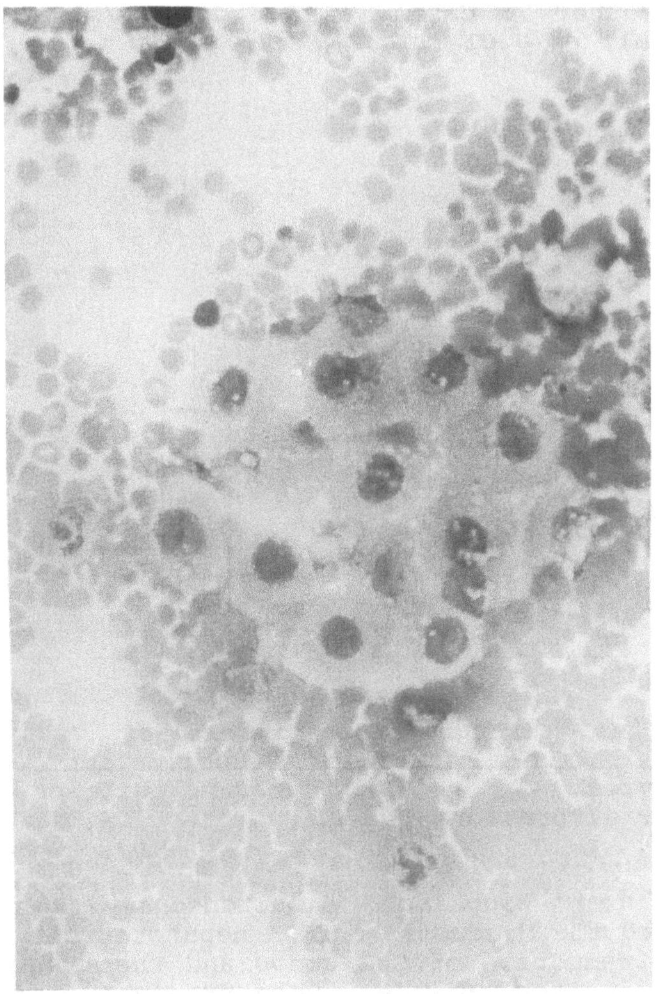

FIG.1 - Isometric vacuolization of the hepatocytes, typical of CSA toxicity.

RESULTS

In 11 FNABs (12.94% of the cases) of 9 patients we observed an isometric vacuolization of the hepatocytes pointing out CSA hepatotoxicity; 8 of these FNABs presented also a concomitant inflammatory cellular infiltrate conditioning a T.C.I. > 3.5 and indicative of acute rejection.

In these 11 cases the trough levels of CSA (measured by RIA kit Sandoz, monoclonal aspecific antibody) were statistically higher than the levels of the other 74 cases: 1520 ± 279 ng/ml vs. 932 ± 467 ng/ml; p< 0.01 (fig.2).

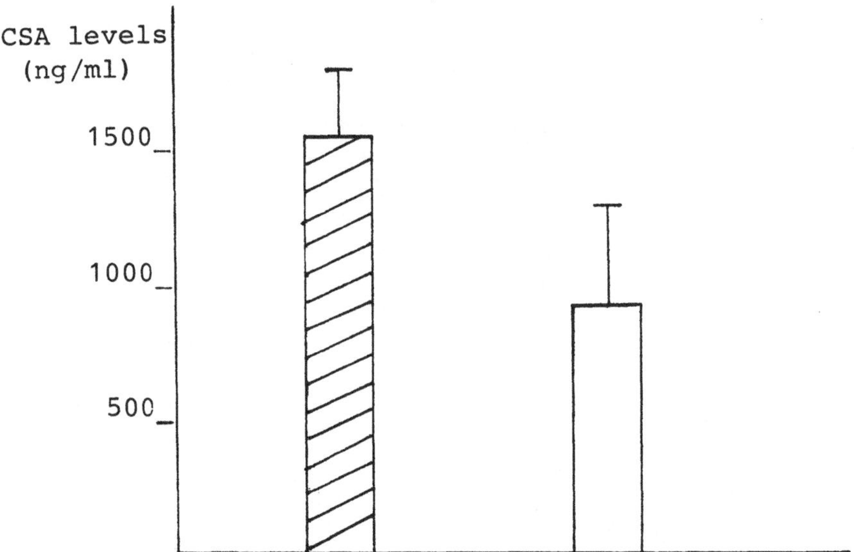

FIG.2 - Trough blood levels of CSA in the patients with isometric vacuolization of the hepatocytes (▧) and in the patients without cellular alterations (□).

7 core biopsies, simultaneously performed, confirmed the diagnosis of CSA hepatotoxicity.

The reduction of CSA doses and the treatment of acute rejection episodes, when present, produced an improvement in liver function and the regression of CSA related cellular lesions.

DISCUSSION

Biochemical parameters of hepatic dysfunction in liver transplanted patients are often aspecific and indicative of different diseases (cholangitis, infections, rejection, cholestasis etc.).

Histological analysis of the liver biopsy is a reliable and early method of diagnosis. In rejection episodes morphological changes appear 4-5 days earlier than biochemical blood markers as the immunologic reaction precedes the tissue damage and the elevation of biochemical parameters.

However liver biopsy is often dangerous and controindicated in case of impaired blood coagulation.

FNAB greatly reduces the complications associated to liver biopsy and evidences the parenchimal damage with a good correlation with transplant histology (4).

Morphological changes of the parenchimal cells, mainly swelling and irregular vacuolization, are present in FNABs during acute rejection episodes with a good correlation with the intensity of inflammation (5).

CSA hepatotoxicity is characterized by an isometric vacuolization of the hepatocytes and the endothelial cells, observed in the FNAB and in the liver biopsy, and often accompagnied by a centrolobular fatty changes and/or centrolobular necrosis.

These morphological changes, due to CSA treatment, are of additional information concerning the target tissue, as for the kidney, and in our series are well correlated with the blood levels of the drug. Hockerstedt et al. (6) didn't find such a correlation, indicating individual differencies in sensitivity to CSA.

These differencies could also be explained by the use of different methods of determination of the blood levels of the drug (CSA alone, CSA and methabolites).

The reversibility of the cellular lesions with the adjustement of the drug doses is well demonstrable and suggests a relationship between hepatotoxicity and blood levels of CSA.

In conclusion we think that the isometric vacuolization of the hepatocytes is a typical and reversible cellular damage caused by the CSA, also observed in renal cells. This damage is clearly identified with the fine-needle aspiration biopsy increasing the diagnostic value of the method. This technique also allows the monitoring of the cellular damage with different dosages of the drug without the complications related to core biopsy.

REFERENCES

1. Hayry P., Willebrand E. von (1981): Am. Clin. Res.,13:288-306.
2. Lautenschlager I., Hockerstedt K., Willebrand E. von, Scheinin T.M., Ahonen J., Scheinin B., Orko R., Kauste A., Eklund B., Salmela K.(1984): Transplant. Proc. 16: 1243-1246.
3. Lautenschlager I., Hockerstedt K., Hayry P. (1991): Transplant. Int. 4: 54-61.
4. Lautenschlager I., Hockerstedt K., Taskinen E., Ahonen J., Korsback C., Salmela K., Orko R., Scheinin B., Scheinin T.M., Hayry P. (1984): Transplantation 38: 330-334.
5. Lautenschlager I., Hockerstedt K., Ahonen J., Eklund B., Isoniemi H:, Korsback C., Petterson E., Salmela K., Scheinin T.M., Willebrand E. von, Hayry P. (1988): Transplantation 46: 47-52.
6. Hockerstedt K., Lautenschlager I., Ahonen J., Eklund B., Korsback C., Makinen J., Pettersson E., Salaspuro M., Scheinin T.M., Willebrand E. von (1988): J. Hepatol. 6: 217-221.

EFFECT OF FK 506 AND CYCLOSPORINS ON MODEL MEMBRANES STUDIED BY NUCLEAR MAGNETIC RESONANCE SPECTROSCOPY

L. Rossaro, S.R. Dowd , V. Simplaceanu , R. Naccarato,
D.H. Van Thiel , and C. Ho

Cyclosporin A (CsA) is a drug that has allowed the field of human organ transplantation to develop from an experimental stage to a practical and effective form of therapy (1). FK 506, a novel compound, is now becoming of interest as an alternative immunosuppressive agent (2, 3), and preliminary reports have appeared to demonstrate its usefulness in organ transplantation (4).

The two drugs are chemically unrelated, yet both suppress T-cell activation by inhibiting mRNA transcription for lymphokines and gamma-interferon (5-10), though the entire mechanism of action remains unclear (11, 12).

Both CsA and FK-506 bind to different cytosolic receptors, cyclophillin (13) and FK-binding protein (14, 15) respectively, with high affinity. These proteins exhibit peptidyl-prolyl isomerase (PPIase) activity which is inhibited by their immunosuppressive ligands, nonetheless the question of whether these proteins and their activities are critically involved in the immunosuppressive action and/or in the side effects of the drugs does not have a definitive answer.

Finally, a common feature of the two agents is their hydrophobicity (2, 16), and their interaction with membrane lipids could possibly play a role in their biological activities associated with signal transduction pathways (12, 17).

D. Galmarini et al. (eds.), Drugs and the Liver: High Risk Patients and Transplantation, 177–184.

We previously reported a study of CsA on model membranes using fluorine-19 nuclear magnetic resonance (^{19}F NMR) spectroscopy (18). This method is particularly useful for investigating the motions and dynamics of a ^{19}F-labeled lipid bilayer in small unilamellar vesicles (SUVs). Its advantage is based on the observation that the ^{19}F NMR resonances arising from the inner and outer leaflets of the bilayer are separated and, following the addition of a drug, it is possible to study lipid-peptide interaction on each leaflet (19). We demonstrated that CsA preferentially sits in the inner leaflet of SUVs, where it affects membrane dynamics and lipid motions. We have now extended those preliminary studies to include different cyclosporin family members, FK 506 and cholesterol.

METHOD

1-Myristoyl-2-(8,8-$^{19}F_2$-difluoromyristoyl)-sn-glycero-3-phosphocholine (^{19}F-DMPC) was synthesized by the method described by Engelsberg et al. (20). Cyclosporins [A (CsA), H (CsH), and G (CsG)] were obtained from Sandoz Ltd. (Basel, Switzerland). FK 506 (Fujisawa Pharmaceutical Co., Ltd, Osaka, Japan) was a gift from Dr. Venkataramman of the University of Pittsburgh.

SUVs were prepared as previously described (18). Separate experiments were performed at different drug concentrations and in some experiments the drugs have been studied with F-labeled SUV, both in the presence and absence of cholesterol (Sigma).

NMR spectra were obtained on a Brüker WH-300 wide-bore spectrometer equipped with an Aspect 2000A computer, operating in the Fourier-transform mode. ^{19}F NMR spectra of the vesicles were obtained at 282.4 MHz with a Brüker high-resolution 5-mm ^{19}F probe. In the experiments evaluating the temperature dependance of the chemical shift, the ^{19}F chemical shifts were referenced to an internal 2-mm capillary containing 10 mM trifluoroacetic acid (TFA) in D_20. In general, 2,000 scans were obtained for each temperature. A spectral width of 11,905 Hz, an acquisition time of 0.344 s (size 8K), a relaxation delay of 2 s, and a 80° pulse of 6 μs were used. Five temperatures ranging from 29° to 49° C, were observed for each experiment.

RESULTS

The effect of temperature on the ^{19}F NMR spectra of ^{19}F-labeled SUV without added drug has previously been reported (18). Two resonances, which arise from the inner and outer leaflets of the bilayer, are seen in the ^{19}F NMR spectra. Changes are observed in the chemical shift values of the control (Figure 1) and in the linewidths of the two resonances as a function of both the temperature and the composition of the SUV. The separation between the two peak positions in the ^{19}F NMR spectrum of ^{19}F-DMPC decreases as the temperature increases. This as a consequence of a down-field shift of the peak from the outer leaflet of the SUV membrane while the position of the inner leaflet resonance remains constant.

When CsA is added at different concentrations (0.4 and 2.0 mol%), the change in the ^{19}F NMR spectra is specific and reproducible. In a dose-dependent manner, the presence of CsA moves the resonance from the inner leaflet of the membrane towards that of the outer leaflet (Figure 1, bottom lines).

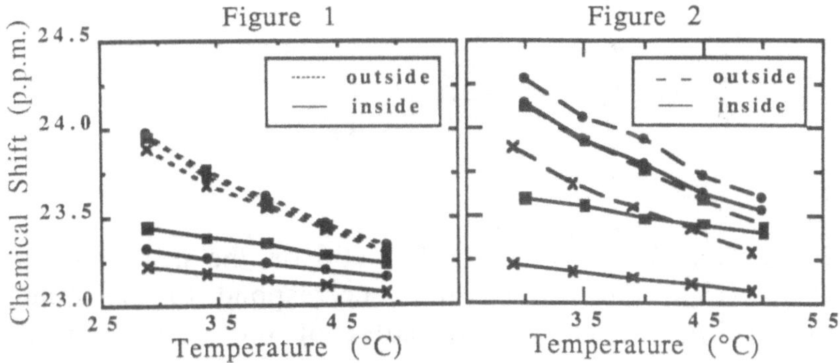

FIGS. 1 and 2. Effect of CsA and CsA+cholesterol on the peak positions of the ^{19}F-SUV. The dotted lines correspond to the outer and the solid lines to the inner leaflet of the vesicle membrane. Symbols: **x** control, Fig. 1: (●) 0.4 mol% and (■) 2.0 mol% CsA; Fig. 2: (●) 3.0 mol% cholesterol + 2.0 mol% CsA and (■) 7.0 mol% cholesterol + 2.0 mol% CsA.

There is no difference in the ^{19}F NMR spectra with and without CsA for the resonance arising from the outside leaflet of the vesicles (Figure 1). When the F-label is in the 4- or 8-position of the acyl chain, a more pronounced effect of concentration and temperature is obtained than when the F-label is in the 12-position (data not shown). Addition of cholesterol to the bilayer leads to a broadening of the resonances and to a shift to higher field. With the addition of a drug, an acceleration of the shift of the inner peak position toward that of the outer is observed (Figure 2).

When the experiments were repeated using CsH and CsG at similar concentrations, the same effect was observed (data not shown). The same was true using FK 506 (Figure 3), with even more effect when cholesterol was present (data not shown), but not when FK 506 was added at low concentrations (Figure 4). The latter finding is relevant since FK 506 is actually used in the clinical situation at a concentration that is 10-100 times less compared to CsA.

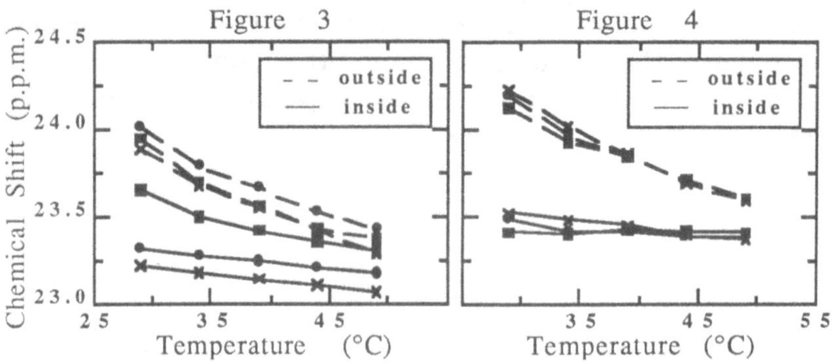

FIGS. 3 and 4. Effect of FK 506 on the peak positions of the ^{19}F-SUV. The dotted lines correspond to the outer and the solid lines to the inner leaflet of the vesicle membrane. Symbols: **x** control, Fig. 3: (●) 0.4 mol% and (■) 2.0 mol% FK 506; Fig. 4: (●) 0.002 mol% and (■) 0.005 mol% FK 506.

DISCUSSION

Cyclosporins which are highly hydrophobic, cyclic undecapeptides, and FK 506, a hydrophobic macrolide, have been studied with F-labeled SUV, both in the presence and absence of cholesterol.

The fluorinated SUV model, studied by ^{19}F NMR, provides a possibility of investigating separately the dynamics of lipids in the inner and in the outer leaflet of the membrane bilayer and their interactions with peptides and other membrane intercalating molecules (19).

The nature of the interaction between CsA and membranes has recently been investigated (16, 21-23). LeGrue et al. (16) have shown that by exposing ^{3}H-labeled CsA to B and T-lymphocytes, kidney cells, and phospholipid vesicles, a similar affinity for binding site and displacement by unlabeled drug was found. O'Leary et al. (21), using calorimetric and spectroscopic techniques on multilayer membranes, found that CsA inserts preferentially into the liquid-crystalline phase without altering lipid structure. Epand et al. (22) using NMR spectroscopy and multilayer liposomes have shown that CsA broadens the ^{31}P NMR spectra suggesting a restriction of the rapid motion of the head groups. As a consequence of this inhibition of the motional freedom of the lipids, a stabilization of the membrane occurs that could account for some of the effect of CsA.

Results from our laboratory (23) on multilayer liposomes show that CsA has a small, but definite effect on the phase transition temperatures of phospholipids labeled with a difluoromethylene group near the head, middle or tail of the acyl chain. Moreover we demonstrated that CsA appears to restrain the motion of the inner lipids of the SUV bilayer membrane (18). These effects demonstrate that CsA disturbs the inner leaflet of the SUV membrane by increasing the order of the lipids. Electron microscopy shows a decrease in the diameter of the SUV with CsA suggesting an effect on the packing of molecules within the bilayer (18). These observations suggest that a perturbation of the membrane function is a result of the partitioning of this hydrophobic molecule into the lipids of the membrane bilayer. These data are further supported by studies on membrane-associated events in human and mouse leukocytes (24, 25).

Our data support the hypothesis that CsA preferentially sit along the acyl chains of phospholipid membranes, in agreement with recent data from Wiedmann et al. (26). Furthermore, CsA appears to be located within the inner layer of SUV (18) suggesting that in vivo similar behavior could occur within the cell. On the other hand it is unlikely that this could explain the entire mechanism of action of CsA, since very similar behavior is shared by other family members such as CsG and CsH, and even by FK 506. It is interesting to note that FK 506, when added at the pharmacological concentrations (i.e. 10-100 time less than CsA dose) (2, 3), has no effect on the model membrane. It is not clear yet if the in vivo observed differences between CsA and FK 506 in terms of effect/concentration ratios simply reflect different rates of absorption and/or metabolism (27).

In conclusion the results suggest that these drugs are present in the membrane. The drugs have a pronounced effect on the structure of the bilayer, causing the inner leaflet to become more ordered and, presumably, to be more densely packed. Added cholesterol broadens both resonances and leads to an even greater packing order when the drugs are added. The evidence of the presence of CsA-sensitive PPIase activity in liver and heart mitochondria closely related to Ca^{2+}-induced non-specific pores in the mitochondrial inner membrane (28, 29) and the preferential packing of the drugs in the inner leaflet of SUV could have relevant implications in relation to the mechanism of action and to the toxicity of both CsA and FK 506 .

REFERENCES

1. Starzl T.E., Weil R., Iwatsuki S., Klintmalm G., Schröter G.P.J., Koep L.J., Iwaki Y., Terasaki P.I. and Porter K.A. (1980): *Surg. Gynecol. Obstet.*, 151: 17-26.
2. Kino T., Hatanaka H., Hashimoto M., Nishiyama M., Goto T., Okuhara M., Kohsaka M., Aoki H. and Imanaka H. (1987): *J. Antibiotics* , 40: 1249-1255.
3. Kino T., Hatanaka H., Miyata S., Inamura N., Nishiyama M., Yajima T., Goto T., Okuhara M., Kohsaka M., Aoki H. and Ochiai T. (1987): *J. Antibiotics* , 40: 1256-1265.
4. Starzl T.E., Todo S., Fung J., Demetris A.J., Venkataramman R. and Jain A. (1989): *Lancet* , 2: 1000-1004.
5. Kronke M., Leonard W.J., Depper J.M., Arya S.K., Wong-

Staal F., Gallo R.C., Waldman T.A. and Greene W.C. (1984): *Proc. Natl. Acad. Sci. USA* , 81: 5214-5218.
6. Herold K.C., Lancki D.W., Moldwin R.L. and Fitch F.W. (1986): *J. Immunol.*, 136: 1315-1321.
7. Granelli-Piperno A. (1990): *J. Exp. Med..*, 171: 533-544.
8. Sawada S., Suzuki G., Kawase Y. and Takaku F. (1987): *J. Immunol.*, 139: 1797-1803.
9. Tocci M.J., Matkovich D.A., Collier K.A., Kwok P., Dumont F., Lin S., Degudicibus S., Siekierka J.J., Chin J. and Hutchinson N.I. (1989): *J. Immunol.*, 143: 718-726.
10. Dumont F.J., Staruch M.J., Koprak S.L., Melino M.R. and Sigal N.H. (1990): *J. Immunol.*, 144: 251-258.
11. Hess A.D. and Colombani P.M. (1986): In: *Progress in Allergy* , edited by J. Borel, pp. 198-221. Karger, Basel.
12. Sigal N.H., Siekierka J.J. and Dumont F.J. (1990): *Biochem. Pharmacol.*, 40: 2201-2208.
13. Handschumacher R.E., Harding M.W., Rice J., Drugge R.J. and Speicher D.W. (1984): *Science* , 226: 544-547.
14. Siekierka J.J., Hung S.H., Poe M., Lin C.S. and Sigal N.H. (1989): *Nature* , 341: 755-757.
15. Harding M.W., Galat A., Uehling D.E. and Schreiber S.L. (1989): *Nature* , 341: 758-760.
16. LeGrue S.J., Friedman A.W. and Kahan B.D. (1983): *J. Immunol.*, 131: 712-718.
17. Szamel M., Berger P. and Resch K. (1986): *J. Immunol.*, 136: 264-269.
18. Rossaro L., Dowd S.R., Ho C. and Van Thiel D.H. (1988): *Transplant. Proc.*, 20: 41-45.
19. Ho C., Dowd S.R. and Post J.F.M. (1985): *Curr. Top. Bioenergetics.*, 14: 53-95.
20. Englesberg M., Dowd S.R., Simplaceanu V., Cook B.W. and Ho C. (1982): *Biochemistry* , 21: 6985-6989.
21. O'Leary T.J., Ross P.D., Lieber M.R. and Levin I.W. (1986): *Biophysical. J.*, 49: 795-801.
22. Epand R.M., Epand R.F. and McKenzie R.C. (1987): *J. Biol. Chem.*, 262: 1526-1529.
23. Dowd S.R., Van Thiel D.H. and Ho C. (1986): *Biophysical. J.*, 49: 306a.
24. Niwa Y., Kano T., Taniguchi S., Miyachi Y. and Sakane T. (1986): *Biochem. Pharmacol.*, 35: 947-951.
25. Matyus L., Balazs M., Aszalos A., Mulhern S. and

Damjanovich S. (1986): *Biochem. Biophys. Acta*, 886: 353-360.
26. Wiedmann T.S., Trouard T., Shekar S.C., Polikandritou M. and Rahman Y-E. (1990): *Biochem. Biophys. Acta*, 1023: 12-18.
27. Thomson A.W. (1989): *Immunol. Today*, 10: 6-9.
28. Halestrap A.P. and Davidson A.M. (1990): *Biochem. J.*, 268: 153-160.
29. Broekemeier K.M. and Pfeiffer D.R. (1989): *Biochem. Biophys. Res. Commun.*, 163: 561-566.

INDEX

Medical Science Symposia Series

1. A. M. Gotto, C. Lenfant, R. Paoletti (eds.) and M. Soma (ass.ed.): *Multiple Risk Factors in Cardiovascular Disease.* 1992 ISBN 0-7923-1938-9
2. A. L. Catapano, A. M. Gotto, Jr., L. C. Smith and R. Paoletti (eds.): *Drugs Affecting Lipid Metabolism.* 1993 ISBN 0-7923-2232-0
3. T. Godfraind, S. Govoni, R. Paoletti and P. M. Vanhoutte (eds.): *Calcium Antagonists. Pharmacology and Clinical Research.* 1993 ISBN 0-7923-2259-2
4. D. Galmarini, L. R. Fassati, R. Paoletti and S. Sherlock (eds.): *Drugs and the Liver: High Risk Patients and Transplantation.* 1993 ISBN 0-7923-2307-6

KLUWER ACADEMIC PUBLISHERS – DORDRECHT / BOSTON / LONDON

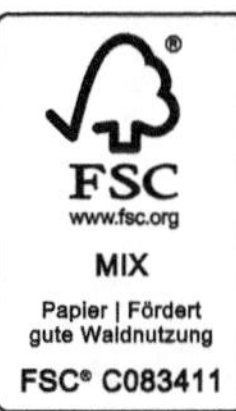

Zeitfracht Medien GmbH
Ferdinand-Jühlke-Straße 7
99095 Erfurt, Deutschland
produktsicherheit@kolibri360.de